Active

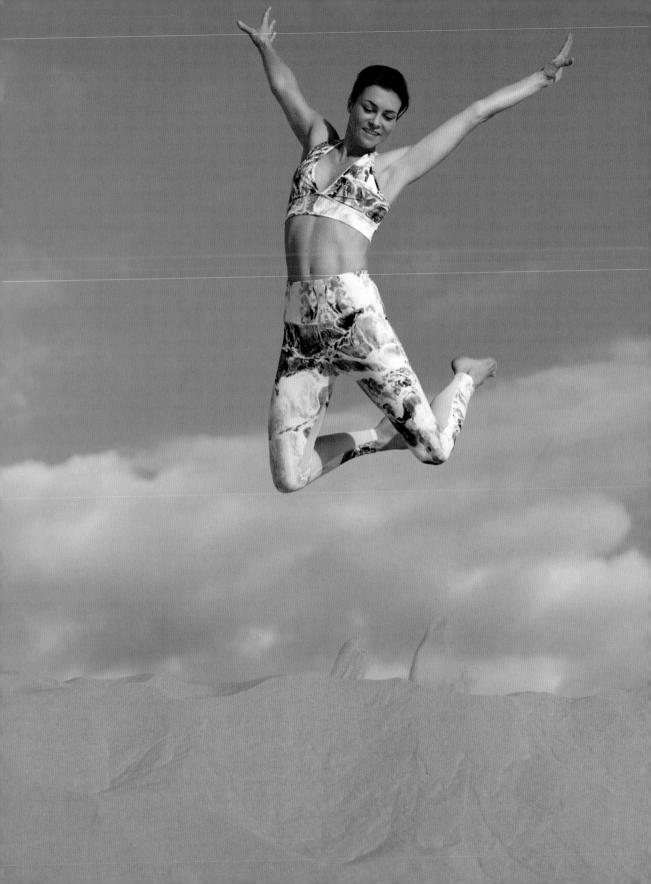

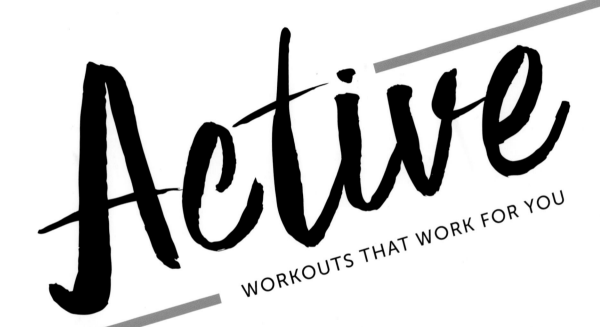

Active

WORKOUTS THAT WORK FOR YOU

HOLLY DAVIDSON

PHOTOGRAPHY BY SEBASTIAN ROOS

KYLE BOOKS

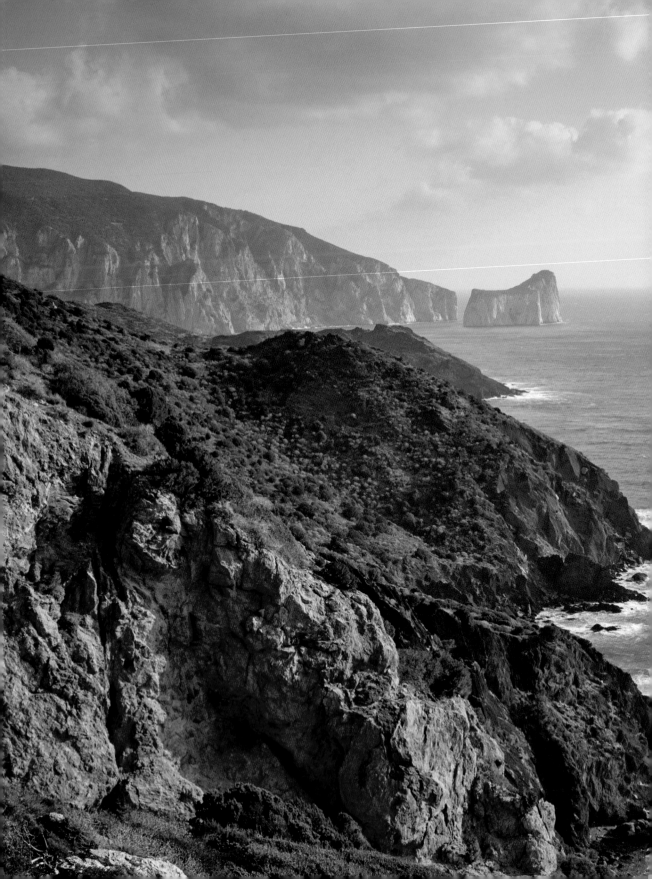

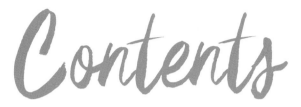

Contents

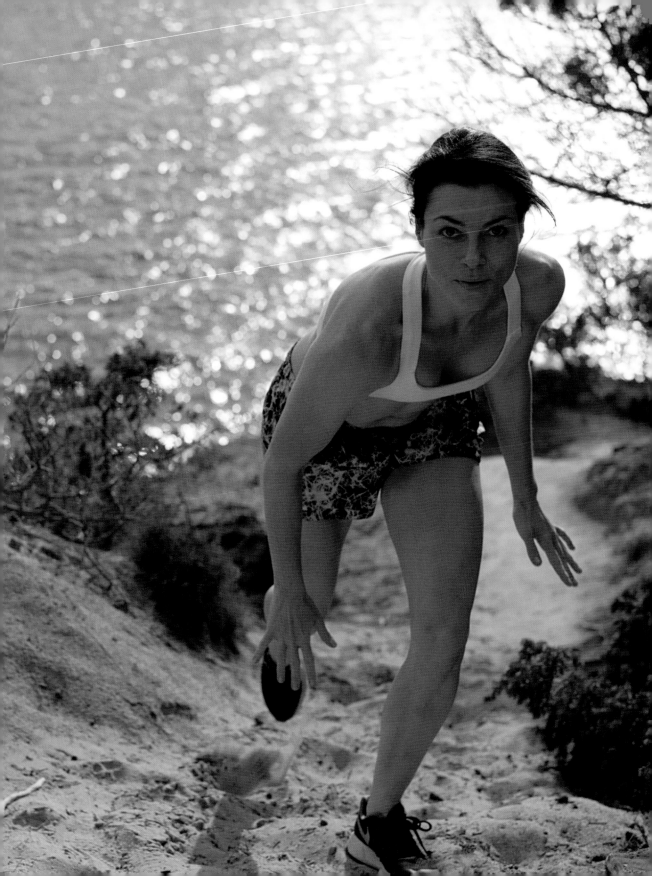

introduction

As children in rural Shropshire, England, my little sister, Jade, and I spent hours adventuring through the countryside, playing in the stream that ran through our garden. We experienced a wonderful sense of freedom and a real passion for being active.

From a young age, I also watched my older sister, Sadie (Frost), develop a successful career in London as a model and actress. I was so inspired by the way she broke into a world that seemed so out of reach to us that, at the age of sixteen, I decided to move to London myself to try and follow in her footsteps. It took a lot of work and a lot of disappointments, but I carved out a good acting career and I loved it.

However, life as an actress comes with its own challenges, like rejection and instability, and in between jobs I grew restless. I began to fill in the gaps with kickboxing, yoga, running and the gym, and found that fitness provided me with a structure and a positive escape. It also gave me a clear mind and a strong body, and reignited that spark that was in me as a child to get active!

In my spare time I began reading about and researching food and the impact it has on our health and wellness. Gradually, as the all-important connections between wholesome cooking and being fit became apparent to me, I decided to leave the exciting but unpredictable world of acting behind and embark on a career as a personal trainer.

Now, a decade on, life has never felt more fulfilling. Each day I get the opportunity to educate and inspire my clients. And so this book is about educating and inspiring you, so you discover a fitness that's compatible with your lifestyle. It's not about overly restrictive diets or too-intense workouts. And it's certainly not about rules. If you set yourself too many rules you're only going to break them.

I believe that the way to get active, be fit and healthy and enjoy exercise is by doing it your way, without any crazy restrictions or fads. Together, we can discover what works for you by implementing small changes that can make a big difference. My approach isn't, 'Go hard or go home'. I prefer encouragement, kindness and support.

Using this book, you can begin to work out wherever is most convenient or comfortable for you, whether that's in your nearest gym, your local park, or even in your own living room. Life is varied, and so are these workouts. Some are more intense than others – some will get your heart racing, muscles burning, and release a real surge of endorphins. Others are there to refresh and restore tired bodies and ease lethargy.

This book is about finding out what works for you, what lights your spark. Sometimes the smallest step in the right direction ends up being the biggest step of your life. So tip-toe if you must, but take that first step...

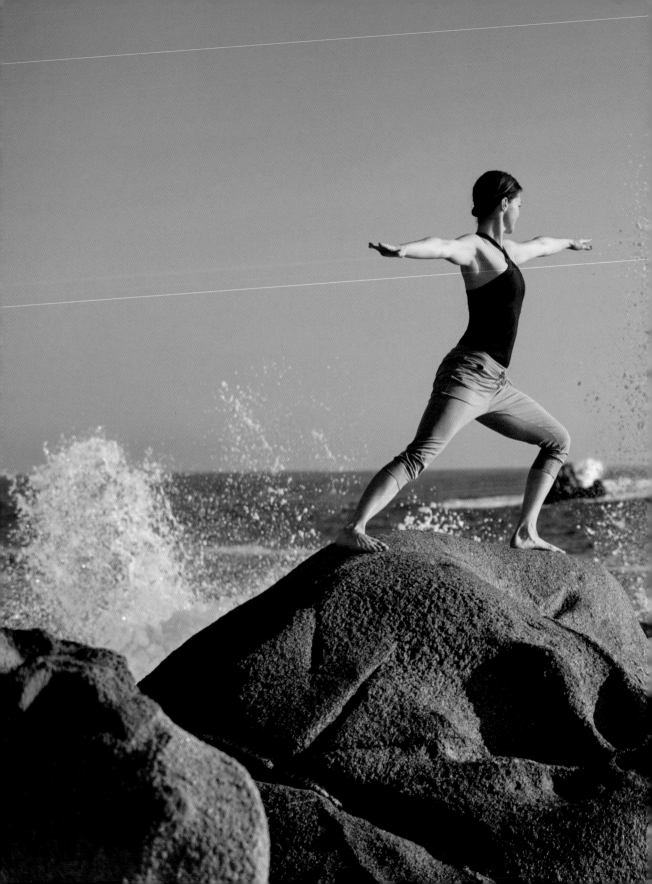

CHAPTER 1

Getting Active

The first step is about addressing your mindset. We live in a fast-paced world where everyone seems to be busy all the time. Too often, exercise slips right down to the bottom of our list of priorities, and there always seems to be an excuse – not enough time, not enough energy, wrong kit, wrong weather. Don't beat yourself up about this – but pay attention to these excuses, and find out what you're really saying. Whether you think you're too short on time, too shy or too old, I'm here to encourage you to have a go. As you make your way through this book, you'll read about the mothers who I train in their living rooms, while their young children play close by, and who go running behind their older children on bikes or take part in fun runs with their husbands, mothers and sisters. Exercise is ageless. So with that in mind, turn the page for my guide to exercising through the ages...

EXERCISING THROUGH THE AGES

YOUR TWENTIES: This decade is a brilliant time for fitness. You're naturally stronger than you were as a teenager. You have good balance, good bone density and plenty of growth hormones that enhance your body's ability to build muscle. Your metabolism is working well and you have the ability to recover quickly from a tough workout, plus you probably have a bit more time on your hands than in your thirties or forties. So use this time to lay down good fitness foundations that will carry you through the decades. Try different classes, sign up for fun runs and join netball, hockey or football clubs to get a sense of the kinds of exercises you like. I loved doing yoga in my twenties too.

YOUR THIRTIES: Your thirties can be a decade when family and work commitments swallow up all your time, and pregnancy (especially repeated pregnancies) also impact on your fitness. But don't forget to pencil in exercise time anywhere you can or fit small bursts of activity into your days. Walk your kids to the park or power walk up hills while pushing a buggy. If you've been doing the same exercises since your twenties, try something new to ensure you're working a good range of muscles as this can help prevent postural problems.

YOUR FORTIES: Pregnancy, hormonal changes and a slowing metabolism can work against you in your forties, but there is still a lot you can do to help yourself. Firstly, go easy on the wine – it's full of sugar and this is the decade where the fight against belly fat really begins. Lift weights regularly to counter this and to preserve your lean muscle mass, which will keep your metabolism fired up. And try to take steps to manage stress. Lots of my forty-something clients are juggling growing children with increasingly demanding careers. Be kind to yourself. Remember to breathe and use exercise as a stress relief (not as a punishment).

YOUR FIFTIES: This is a time to focus on your core, so try Pilates and yoga. You may feel a little more achy in your joints, but don't let this put you off exercise and simply adapt your moves accordingly. Look after your heart with daily walks and anything that gets you moving and sweating, like gardening and keep-fit classes. The most important thing is to just keep moving!

YOUR SIXTIES: Keep moving every day, keep lifting weights (even light ones) and try to do a little yoga or Pilates every week to keep your bones strong, your core healthy and to prevent that slippery slope to frailty and feeling old before your time.

YOUR SEVENTIES AND BEYOND: There is simply no cut-off point when it comes to exercise. You see seventy- and eighty-somethings taking part in marathons, half marathons and fun runs and out walking or hiking. Even gardening or walking your dog counts, so just keep active and, as always, do what you love. The happiest, healthiest people simply carry on moving, but in a way that suits them and their changing bodies.

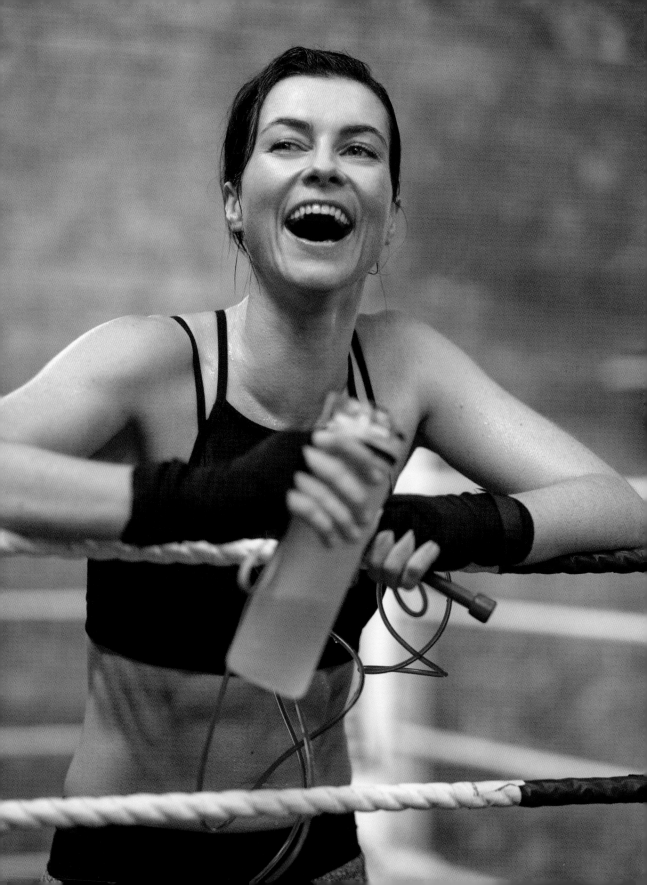

'BUT I DON'T HAVE ANY TIME'

Time can be a big stumbling block when it comes to exercise and I'm often told by new clients that they just 'don't have time'. Women in particular seem to put themselves and their needs right at the bottom of their to-do lists, behind children, jobs, household chores and life admin. But you can't look after everything else if you're not looking after yourself! Remember the saying, 'You can't pour from an empty cup'.

The good news is, time doesn't have to be a barrier to fitness. If you're waiting for a point in your life when you think you'll have enough time for exercise, you'll end up waiting a long time. Life is busy and will always be busy – you just have to find ways to fit exercise into your life right now and bump it (and therefore yourself) further up that to-do list, even if it means letting something else slip down occasionally.

New clients will often tell me that they don't have time to get fit because they work long hours, travel a lot for work or have young children. They tell me they hardly have a minute to spare and I'm sure you've told yourself this before. But you do. After all, if you spend five minutes browsing Facebook when you wake up, then you have five minutes to do a bit of yoga or stretching on your bedroom floor.

Fitness isn't about hour-long sessions in a gym that's a twenty-minute drive from your house. Fitness is right there in your bedroom from the moment you wake up. Anybody can get fit – you just have to make that choice.

A lack of confidence can also be another barrier to fitness (if you let it). And perhaps, when you say you don't have time to get fit, it's really because you don't have the confidence to try. And I get that. Sometimes it's simpler to persuade yourself that you don't have time as then you don't have to face your fears about how you look in exercise clothes or how you'll keep up in a gym class.

But this is your journey. It's tempting to compare ourselves to other women in the gym, at the office or on the school run, or to women with different body shapes, genetics and lifestyles to our own. Or worse, to social media, where glossy, edited snapshots of other people's lives compare so unfavourably with our own reality. Even I struggle with seeing other personal trainers on social media

Identify your time drain

Even those of us who feel like we live incredibly busy lives have 'time drains' – habits and behaviour patterns that eat up precious minutes without us realising. Social media is a big one. So here's a challenge: think about what your time drain is and, for one day, add up how many minutes you lose to it. Five minutes on Facebook here, a quick scroll through Twitter there – it all adds up. Sometimes seeing the total figure for that day's time drain can be a bit of a revelation. You might find you're actually losing a whole half hour to it (or even more). Of course, we all need down time. But a gentle workout can be a far more effective use of down time than living vicariously through someone else's Instagram feed.

who might look fitter, stronger and in better workout gear than me. But I know to be kind to myself and so I simply put down my phone, pop my headphones in and go for a run in the park because I know that all that really matters is my own fitness journey. I feel great when I exercise and I can't imagine a life without it, so what anybody else is doing doesn't really matter at all.

So if you take the time – and remember, you only need a little time – to get fit, everything else in your life will feel easier. You'll feel fitter, stronger, happier, you'll sleep better and you'll have more concentration. And don't you deserve that? When I haven't exercised in a while I feel half as good as usual. So don't go through life only feeling half as good as your full potential.

Over the coming chapters I'm going to be showing you how to get fit during a busy working week. Whether you have ten minutes or an hour, whether you join a gym, do a bit of yoga on your bedroom floor or head to your local park with your kids, this is exercise you can fit into your day – all of the workouts are short and easy to incorporate into a busy schedule. Very few of my clients have the luxury of lots of time because they work, travel or they're parents, so they often have to fit their fitness in around their busy lives. I'm going to show you how – and where – you can sneak it in.

TABITHA, 30, PUBLISHING ASSISTANT

'I never really enjoyed PE at school, and even as an adult I felt quite self-conscious about exercising. I always found excuses not to do it and the main excuse, and one I know a lot of my friends make too, is that I didn't have enough time. However, I also knew that I needed to start taking better care of myself and, after speaking to Holly, I realised that it was time to start being more honest with myself and to make time in my day to fit exercise in.

'I had a bad habit of hitting the snooze button on my alarm several times each morning before dragging myself out of bed. However, these days, I plug my phone in to charge on the other side of the room, which means I have to get out of bed in order to turn off the alarm. Once I'm out of bed, I don't feel the need to crawl back in and I use that extra time each morning to do a yoga workout.

'I also joined a swimming pool that's really close to my office and I go swimming every day in my lunch break. Before this, I would have told you that I didn't have time to take a proper lunch break, and I'd always eat my lunch hunched over my desk. However, getting out of the office and exercising means I come back to my desk refreshed and energised. Plus, I get more work done in this state than I ever did by slogging through the whole day without a break.

'The best part is, once I started making time for fitness, I realised how much I enjoy it – and not just the benefits, but the exercise itself.'

START SMALL

I believe the biggest obstacle to getting fit is our mindset. So many of us set ourselves up for failure by simply thinking we can't do something (we can!). And the key to switching this mindset is to start small. When I first started to write this book it felt like a huge, overwhelming task. 'Where do I even begin?' I kept thinking, which is what clients say when they first come to see me.

Exercise should be about becoming stronger, fitter, more energised, sleeping better and feeling less stressed

---

So I told myself what I tell them – don't see getting fit as one big huge goal. Don't think, 'I need to lose two stone and become super fit'. Don't think you need to join a £100-a-month gym and find the time to go five times a week. Don't think you need to stop eating chocolate and drinking wine immediately and just live on salad. Stop panicking and over-planning and just start small. Simply break down your goals into small, doable chunks and then slowly, and comfortably, work your way through them. For me, that meant taking this book chapter by chapter. Paragraph by paragraph. For you, that might mean doing three walks a week or going shopping and buying yourself a new gym kit. (I'm going to talk more about that later, because it's always a good place to start and gets you in the right zone.)

ASK YOURSELF WHY YOU'RE DOING THIS

Don't think in terms of pounds lost or dress sizes dropped (although that will happen). Think in terms of how you feel. Exercise should be about becoming stronger, fitter, more energised, sleeping better, feeling less stressed with our friends and family, digesting our food better and having more confidence, mental alertness and concentration. It's about feeling great rather than exhausted when you wake up, and having a strong, lean, fit body that feels capable and strong, rather than old, sluggish and creaky before its time. Best of all, feeling better physically is one of the first benefits you'll notice when you start getting more active – you don't need to wait long for this reward.

The other problem with the motivation of losing weight just to look good is that it often comes with a sell-by date. For example, if you eat really well and go to the gym in the lead-up to a holiday or wedding, there's a tendency to let all the good work slide when the holiday is over. There's this 'on again, off again' mentality to dieting and exercise when really, eating well and moving your body regularly should be a way of life and not part of a six-week plan.

I say, get fit for life, not just a bikini !

However, I do appreciate that weight loss is also a goal for many people who want to get fit and, if you're carrying excess weight, that's completely fine. It's OK to want to look better in your clothes; it just shouldn't be your only or main goal. If you have a week where you don't lose any weight or your tummy is still a little bigger than you'd like it to be, you can still pat yourself on the back for feeling more energised or less stressed or for improving your sleep.

LET MUSIC HELP YOU

Have a good playlist at the ready as some very good studies show that music can help you work out for longer and more efficiently. For example, researchers from Brunel University in the UK found that exercise performance improved by up to 15 per cent when the study participants listened to music during a workout. As well as improving performance, the researchers also found that listening to music lowered the perception of effort (i.e. the participants didn't notice quite how hard they were working when they were listening to music). And then of course, music can help lift your mood and get you 'in the zone'. I know that listening to really upbeat tracks helps me focus and keep a really good pace when I'm running around my local roads.

The Olympic swimmer Michael Phelps famously listened to fast-paced music on his headphones right before a race. 'I have walked out to race with my headphones on throughout my whole career and listen to music until the last possible moment,' he told an interviewer after winning six gold medals at the 2005 Athens Olympics. 'It helps me to relax and get into my own little world.'

So think about which of your favourite songs will motivate you to exercise and help you get moving.

SILVIA, 45, SOFTWARE TESTER AND MUM OF TWO

'About two years ago, a friend recommended Holly to me. Back then, I was at work for half the week, and the other half I was working from home and looking after my two children, who are now seven and eleven.

'For the first half of the week, when I was at work, I was fairly healthy. But I spent the rest of the week, like a lot of mums, rushing around, meeting the kids' needs but not really looking after my own. I just wanted to feel fitter and healthier and, when I first met Holly and she asked me what my goal was, I told her I wanted to learn how to run.

'I had signed up for a 5k with a friend, but I was starting to think that I should pull out because I couldn't run very far without getting out of breath. However, thanks to Holly, I ran that 5K only six weeks later. She helped me overcome all my fears. I was so scared of getting out of breath or even fainting in public, but Holly showed me how to regulate my breathing and keep calm. She made me see that I had to take the pressure off myself – if I needed to stop and walk, I could. I realised that I was running this race for me, not to break any records, not to beat anyone else, but to prove to myself that I had the confidence to try. And getting to the finishing line was the best thing ever.

'That was two years ago and since then I've completed three half-marathons. If I can do it, anybody can.'

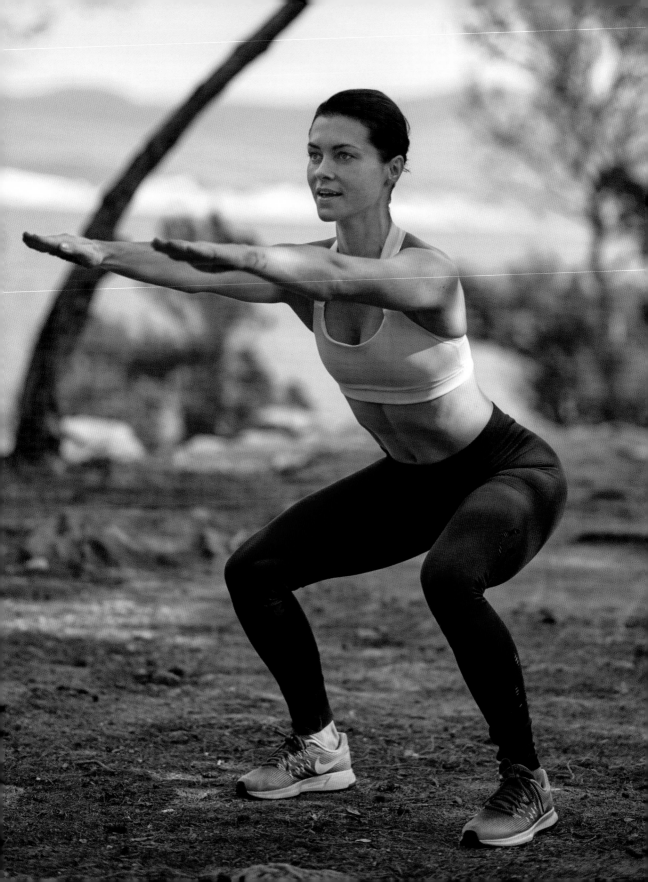

GET THE RIGHT KIT

You don't have to spend a fortune; most high-street shops now have a fitness section where you can pick up gym leggings, tops, exercise bras and trainers for a reasonable price. Or look in your own wardrobe – are there any long-forgotten gym leggings and a T-shirt lying around? Anyway, here's a quick guide to dressing for success.

A GOOD PAIR OF LEGGINGS

Invest in a nice pair of exercise leggings that will support your body and flatter your shape (regular leggings often show off more than you might intend to, especially after a few wears!). You can either buy these from the major fitness brands, like Nike, Adidas or Reebok, from premium fitness brands, like Sweaty Betty and Lululemon, or from high-street shops, like Gap Active, Marks & Spencer or Topshop. Shop around and see what you like and what you can afford.

A WELL-FITTED SPORTS BRA

This is non-negotiable. If you're confident about your bra size, buy a good supporting sports bra in your usual size, making sure you try it on first. Or ask to be fitted properly (many high-street shops offer this service, so ask). A poorly fitting sports bra can lead to breast tissue damage, so it's vital to get this right.

TRAINERS

Again, you can buy these from a big brand or the high street, but it's best to get advice when buying to make sure you get the best pair to suit your feet and your gait. Many running shops have a free in-store fitting service to help you make the right choice. Your trainers are a real investment, so do your research now rather than risk injury later. As a general rule, trainers need to be replaced every 500 miles (which is roughly every year if you're a fairly regular exerciser, or sooner if you run a lot).

TOPS AND T-SHIRTS

A lot of this is down to personal style, but I would recommend a proper dry-fit sports top for comfort and ease of movement.

TAKING THOSE FIRST STEPS

So, once you've got your kit and your playlist ready, it's time to put your trainers on and begin. If you're completely new to fitness, aim to go for three 20-minute walks a week. If you're fairly fit, make them fast-paced walks that get you almost out of breath and, if you're a little fitter, go for three gentle jogs. Don't be tempted to go all out and run as fast and as hard as you can. Just start small and slow, but crucially, build on it. Don't simply go for three leisurely walks, week after week. Push yourself a little bit harder each time by turning a walk into a power walk, a power walk into a run, and so on. If you begin to feel a buzz and want to go for 30 minutes, do it. If you're worn out after 20 minutes, congratulate yourself for taking that first step and head home feeling proud. And if you find yourself really enjoying running, the 'Couch to 5k' app (iTunes) is a great aid to get you started and build up your fitness.

Move your body more in other ways, too – potter about at home rather than watch TV or browse on your phone, and walk briskly up and down stairs as much as you can. Walk up (and down) a moving escalator. Go for a little walk at lunchtime, finding places you've never been to before. I can't emphasise enough the huge impact all these little activities can have on your health.

Walking is one of the greatest forms of exercise because it works a huge number of muscles, it's free, easy and comes with a very low risk of injury. It also involves moving your body in the exact way it was designed to move. Humans aren't supposed to sit all day long – they're designed to walk. So walk as much as you can and, if you feel fit enough, supercharge your walk by putting on some trainers, picking up the pace and keeping your arms at right angles (so your fists are just below your chest) as this burns more calories and boosts fitness. Try to move more in your everyday life and you'll reap huge health rewards – as I was writing this, a new study from the University of Cambridge found that a 20-minute walk every day cuts your risk of premature death by almost a third.

Take away the negative associations and find an exercise you like.

As well as walking, try a fitness class at your local gym or one of the exercise routines in this book. Experiment a little to see if you like it and, if not, try something else. This is really important because, if you enjoy exercise, you'll stick at it. Don't ever see exercise as a punishment for something you ate. Or just as a means to lose weight. Or as something you 'should do'.

Take away the negative associations and find an exercise you like. I love running, but I know it's not for everybody. It gives me such a buzz, clears my head and I love the freedom of just heading out the door for a really good run around the streets or through the park in the fresh air. But I have friends who can't stand it. They find it boring, or lonely, or hard on their joints. And to those friends I say, 'Don't run!'. If you don't enjoy something, don't do it. It's that simple. Ask yourself what you do like. Do you like dancing fitness classes? Or yoga? How about kickboxing? Or a bit of all three, in which case mix and match your fitness.

As ever, this is your journey, so if you're the kind of person who likes to set goals and chart your progress, then get a fitness tracker that can help motivate you with prompts and alerts. Some trackers also track sleep, heart rate and many other things, and enable you to monitor all the changes your body is going through. However, if you're not keen on technology or if you're the kind of person who may feel bad and beat themself up a little after a fairly inactive day, then leave these well alone. Getting fit is about doing what works for you.

Do you like exercising alone or with friends? I have clients who work all day in busy offices and like to work out alone where they don't have to talk to anybody else and can just have a moment to themselves for the first time all day. But I have other clients who are home all day with young children and enjoy being around others, so for them a sociable gym class is the best option.

How do you feel about your body? If you feel self-conscious about how you look or how well you can keep up in a class, then maybe go to the gym at an off-peak time or start with a home workout. It's about making exercise work for you, rather than forcing yourself to do something you feel uncomfortable with. It can be daunting when you first start, especially if you're not overly confident about your body, but believe me nobody is looking at you. They are there to get fit themselves and anyway, you're not doing this for anybody else, you're doing it for you.

If a gym class feels too much, try working out at home first (see Chapter 2, At Home).

Or try a fitness DVD or work out with a friend, perhaps going for a jog in the evenings or first thing on a Saturday. It's best to pick a friend who's roughly the same level of fitness as you – maybe a little fitter, maybe a little less so. But don't go with somebody a lot fitter than you as you may feel self-conscious if you can't keep up and then you'll be tempted to cancel.

Lastly, all the exercise routines in this book work the whole body. Clients often ask me for an exercise that will target their wobbly tummy or upper arms. But I tell them that in order to target these areas, they need

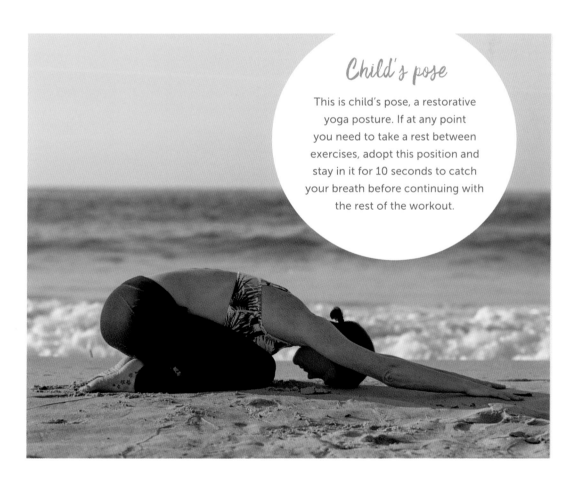

Child's pose

This is child's pose, a restorative yoga posture. If at any point you need to take a rest between exercises, adopt this position and stay in it for 10 seconds to catch your breath before continuing with the rest of the workout.

to work the whole body. Another reason is time – you'll get better results in less time by working your whole body at once. I'm not a big believer in working your arms one day and your abs the next, because if you're feeling run down the next day or your child's poorly, then you'll miss a whole body part. It's far better to blitz your whole body every time.

You'll get better results in less time by working your whole body at once

---

The workouts in this book will help you explore the many different places and ways in which we can all enjoy exercise. Some will get your heart pumping, others will tone and stretch and some will focus on posture. They can be adapted to suit all levels of fitness and ability and you can pick and choose what you do so that everything easily fits around your busy life and follows the ebb and flow of how you feel, whether you're full of energy and want to get your heart racing, or you need to get grounded after a stressful week.

GIVE YOURSELF A BREAK (BUT ONLY A SMALL ONE!)

This is really important because you need to listen to your body and acknowledge how you're feeling and allow for the changing patterns of life. Sometimes you'll have a cold, it will be raining outside, your children will be off school with a bug, or you just won't feel like exercising. In these situations, don't put pressure on yourself – just accept it. However, don't keep making excuses, otherwise your

new habit of exercise will soon be replaced by the old habit of not exercising. But know that it's OK to skip it occasionally. Don't beat yourself up over it.

Lastly, don't compare yourself to anybody else. Social media is a wonderful thing at times. I use it and love following different fitness experts and bloggers for ideas and inspiration, but there's a tipping point and you should never look at anybody else's body, or diet, or weight and compare it to your own.

So remember this; fitness is everywhere and getting fit isn't a mountain to climb – it's a simple staircase. And you can climb it one step at a time.

HOW STRONG IS YOUR PELVIC FLOOR?

If you've had children or have a weak pelvic floor, you may have problems with skipping or jumping and feel like you're going to wet yourself during a workout. Don't worry! It just means you need to strengthen your pelvic floor, which is a muscle like any other.

Your pelvic floor is a hammock of muscles and the primary stabiliser of your stomach muscles. I tell all my new mum clients to work theirs soon after giving birth, but it's never too late to work yours. They're the muscles you would clench to stop yourself peeing mid-flow. So work them regularly when you have an empty bladder (not when you actually need to pee) and do 10 or 20 clenches several times throughout the day.

Another good exercise for your pelvic floor is this: Start on all fours with your back straight. Take a deep breath in and let your tummy fill up with air and drop it to the floor.

Then slowly breathe out and draw your belly button in towards your spine and squeeze your pelvic floor muscles at the same time.

ARE YOU USING YOUR CORE?

Before you begin any exercise, it's a very good idea to think about your core. By this I mean the corset of muscles surrounding the back and abdomen, which are so important for keeping our bodies stable and balanced, supporting the spine and therefore protecting against injury. In my line of work, I see so many injuries caused by people doing normal everyday activities, like turning back to see to their kids in the car, reaching up high for something in a cupboard or leaning into the car boot and taking out suitcases. We don't realise how all these bending and lifting and twisting movements place a load on our spine and, if we don't provide it with additional support by engaging our core, we leave our bodies very vulnerable to strains and injuries. Here's a quick test that will immediately tell you if you're good at engaging your core, or if you need to work on it some more.

THE STRING TEST

Place a heavy-ish object, such as a water bottle on the floor in front of you. Stand up straight and draw your stomach in (don't

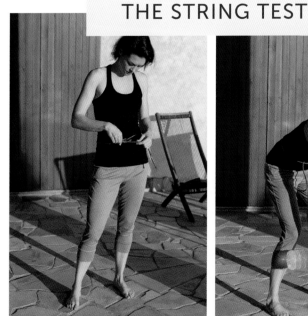

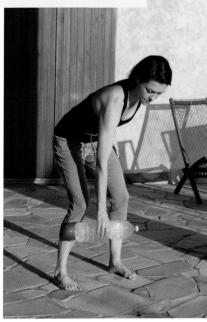

suck it in). It should feel as if the deep core muscles are slightly tightening. Tie a piece of string around your waist (so it goes over your belly button). You should be able to feel the string around you but it shouldn't pinch. Now pick up the object.

Does your tummy press against the string when you bend? If it does, this indicates that you are relaxing your tummy muscles when picking up a heavy load, which can put extra strain on your back.

Exercise often imitates life. That's why we do it – to make everyday chores easier. It's therefore extremely important that we exercise consciously with good form.

The workouts

Every chapter in this book contains workouts suited to different environments. For every workout, I've given you a rough idea of how long the whole thing will take, so you know how much time to set aside. The exact time will vary from person to person, but it's a useful rough guide. On pages 168–170 you'll find summaries of every workout, for an easy at-a-glance guide.

The rest of this chapter is devoted to warm ups, cool downs and stretches for you to use alongside the workouts.

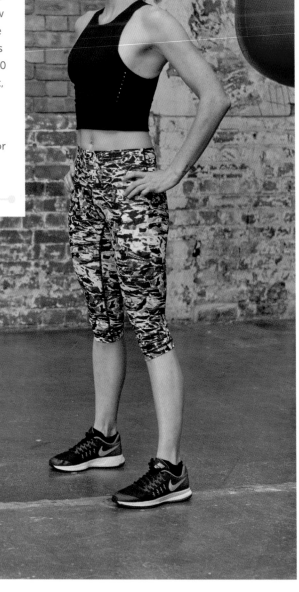

1

2

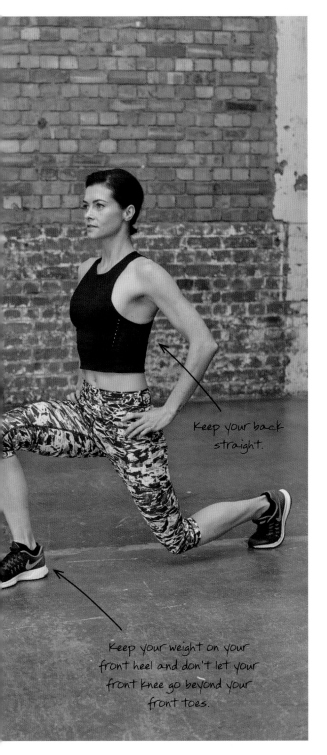

Keep your back straight.

Keep your weight on your front heel and don't let your front knee go beyond your front toes.

WARMING UP

Warming up before any kind of exercise is so important. Why? Because as well as getting your head in the right place for exercise, a good warm-up also warms up (hence the name!) your muscles, which will help prevent injury. The following is a great full-body warm-up that could also be used as a mini workout if you're new to exercise, short on time or just feel like your body needs a quick once-over.

Repeat each action for 60 seconds before moving on to the next.

- - - - - - - - - - - - - - - -
6 minute warm-up

WALKING LUNGES

HOW TO DO IT: Stand tall, core engaged, with your feet hip-width apart.

With your right leg, take a big step forwards into the lunge position, so both your knees are at right angles. Your back knee should be as close to the floor as possible.

Push off the back foot and take a big lunge forwards with the left leg so you repeat the move on the other side. **{60 seconds}**

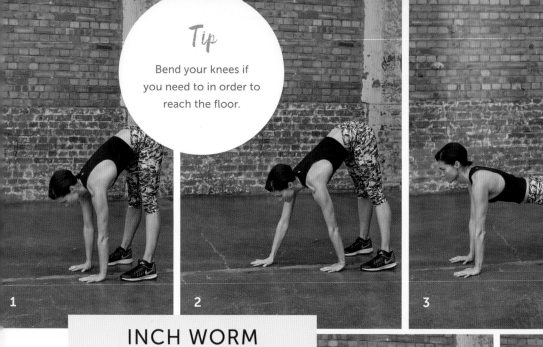

Tip

Bend your knees if you need to in order to reach the floor.

1

2

3

INCH WORM

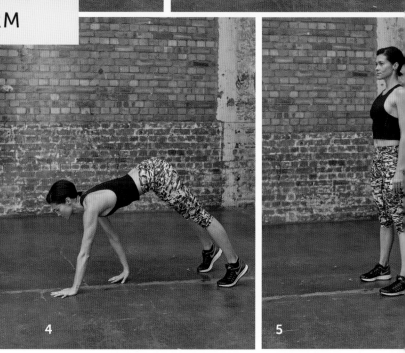

4

5

HOW TO DO IT: Stand tall, core engaged, with your feet hip-width apart. Hinge at the hips until you can place your hands on the floor. Slowly walk your hands forwards until you're in a raised plank position. Hold for a moment. Slowly walk your hands back and return to standing. **{60 seconds}**

Tip

Holding this for 60 seconds can be quite tough on the arms, so remember to take a break in child's pose (page 19) if you need to.

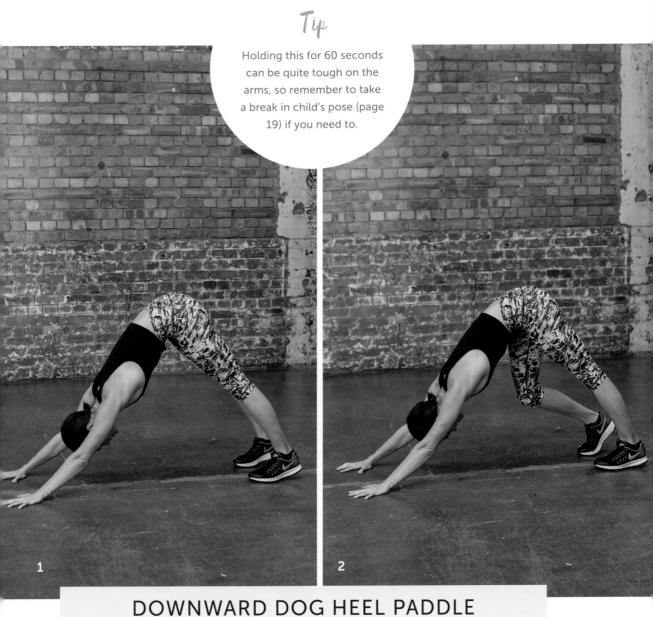

1

2

DOWNWARD DOG HEEL PADDLE

HOW TO DO IT: Get into a downward dog position as shown – hands shoulder-width apart, feet hip-width apart and your hips up and back to form an 'A' shape. Engage your core and relax your upper back. Keep your head and neck relaxed.

Bend your right knee and lift your right heel, keeping the ball of the foot on the floor. Repeat on the other leg in a pedalling motion. **{60 seconds}**

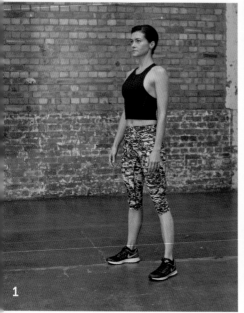

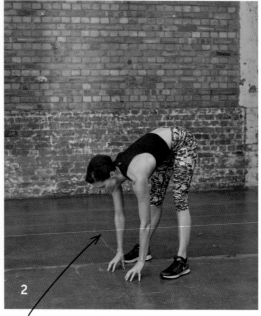

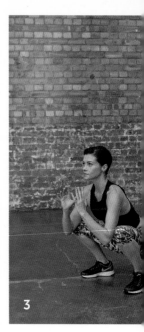

Don't worry if you can't touch the floor – just reach as far as you can.

Your shoulders should be directly over your wrists, arms straight, and your body in one straight line, from shoulders to heels.

PLANK TO LUNGE ROTATION

HOW TO DO IT: Start in a high plank position.

Take a big step forwards with your right foot, placing it on the outside of your right hand. Now reach your right hand upwards, rotating your torso to do so.

Rotate the torso back to neutral, return your hand to the floor, step back into a plank position and repeat with the left side.

{60 seconds}

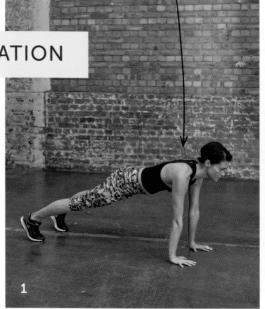

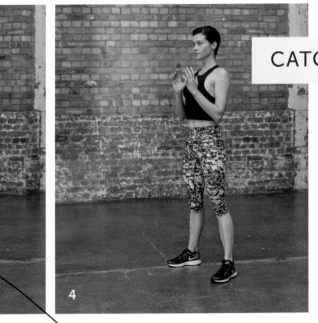

4

CATCHER SQUAT TO STAND

HOW TO DO IT: Stand tall, core engaged, with your feet hip-width apart. Hinge forwards at the hips and touch the floor.

Now bend your knees into a low squat and place your hands to your chest as if you were about to catch a ball. Come back up to standing by pressing your heels into the floor, keeping your chest lifted. **{60 seconds}**

If you can't get your heels flat on the floor in this position, place a rolled-up towel under them for support. You can keep it there throughout.

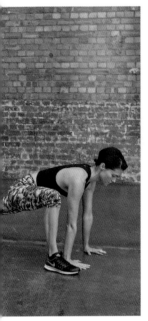

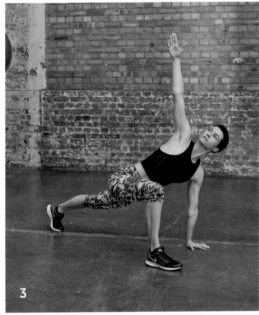

3

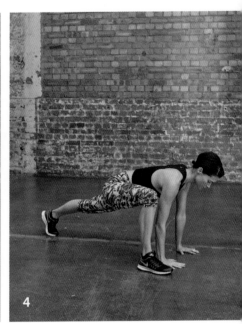

4

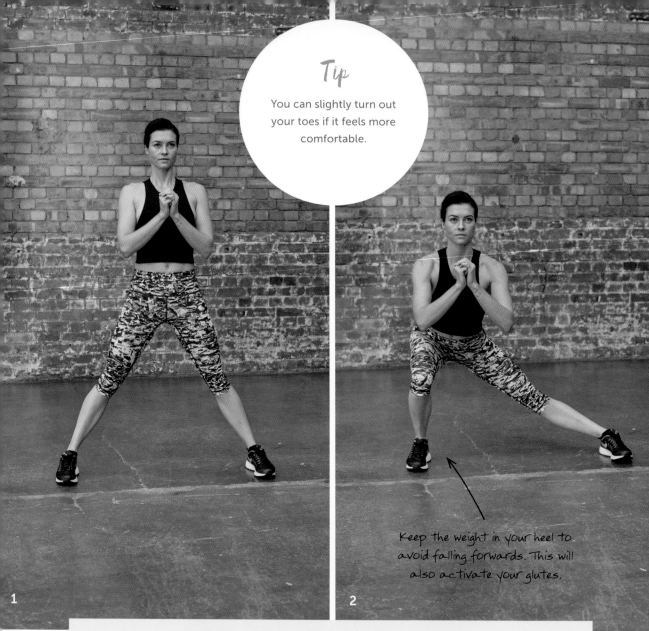

Tip

You can slightly turn out your toes if it feels more comfortable.

Keep the weight in your heel to avoid falling forwards. This will also activate your glutes.

1

2

LOW SIDE-TO-SIDE LUNGE

HOW TO DO IT: Stand tall, core engaged, with your feet wide apart.

Bend your right knee and lean your weight to that side, keeping the other leg straight. Try to get as low as possible.

Push off the heel to return to standing and then move your weight to the other side in a flowing movement. **{60 seconds}**

POSTURE WARM-UP

This is an alternative warm up. It's zero impact on joints, so if you're new to exercise this is a gentle, focussed introduction, but it's also great for the more advanced exerciser to reset and mobilise

----

5 minute warm-up

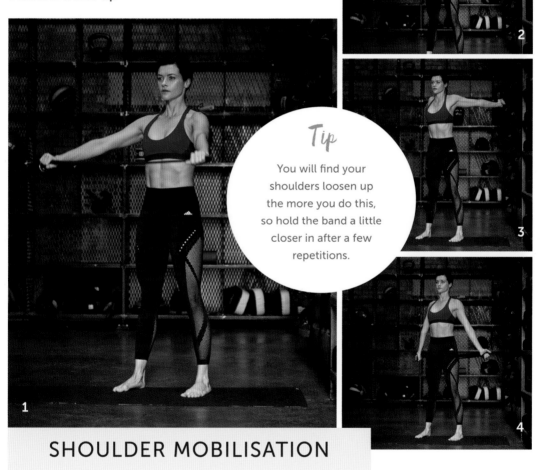

> *Tip*
>
> You will find your shoulders loosen up the more you do this, so hold the band a little closer in after a few repetitions.

SHOULDER MOBILISATION

HOW TO DO IT: Stand tall, core engaged, and hold a resistance band, a skipping rope or even the tie from your dressing gown with one end in each hand. Hold it wide enough so you can rotate your arms fully behind and in front of you, keeping your arms straight. **{10 reps}**

CAT AND COW

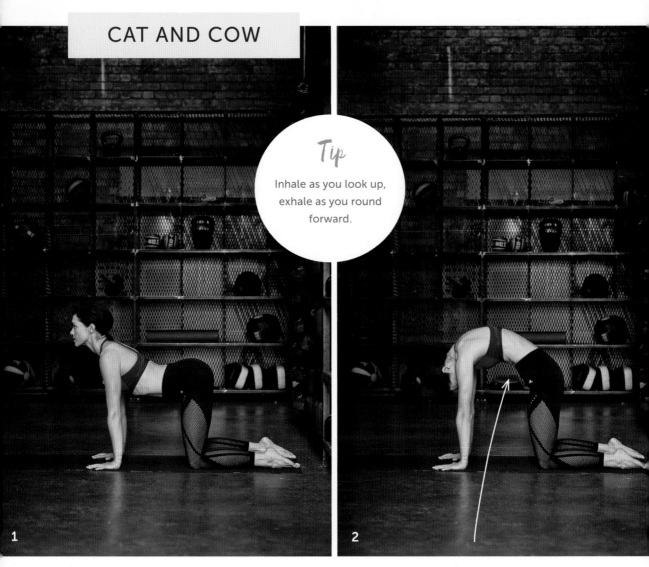

Tip

Inhale as you look up, exhale as you round forward.

Really feel you're sucking your stomach in and up for this movement.

HOW TO DO IT: Start on all fours with hands under shoulders and knees under hips.

Lift your head and look up while arching your spine and letting your stomach relax towards the floor.

Reverse the move by tucking your chin in to your chest and rounding your spine to the sky, drawing your stomach in. **{10 reps}**

THORACIC ROTATION

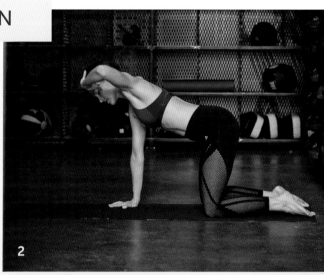

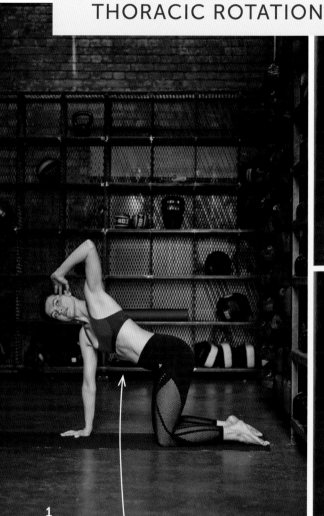

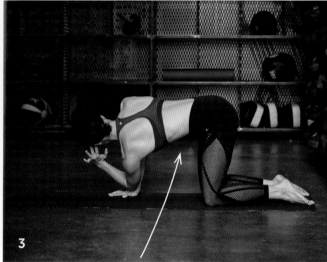

Keep your core tight throughout.

Don't allow your lower back to overarch.

HOW TO DO IT: Start on all fours with hands under shoulders and knees under hips.
Place one hand on the back of your head, rotating your body to the side as you reach the bent elbow up to the sky. Now rotate back down, moving your bent elbow towards the opposite wrist. Repeat on the other side. **{5 reps each side}**

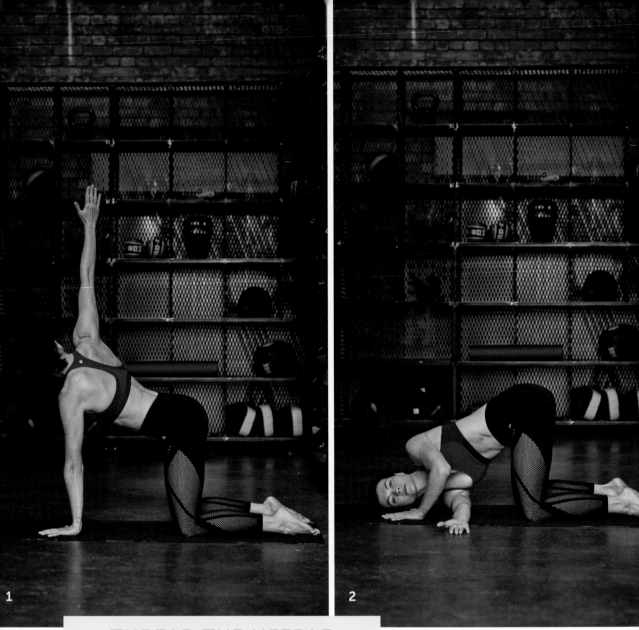

1

2

THREAD THE NEEDLE

HOW TO DO IT: Start on all fours with hands under shoulders and knees under hips. Reach your right arm towards the sky, opening up as far as you can. Now thread this arm through the gap between your left hand and knee, bending your left elbow. If possible, continue the threading movement until your right shoulder and ear touch the floor. Return to the previous position with your arm reaching towards the sky. Complete 5 reps, then do the other side. **{5 reps each side}**.

ACTIVE

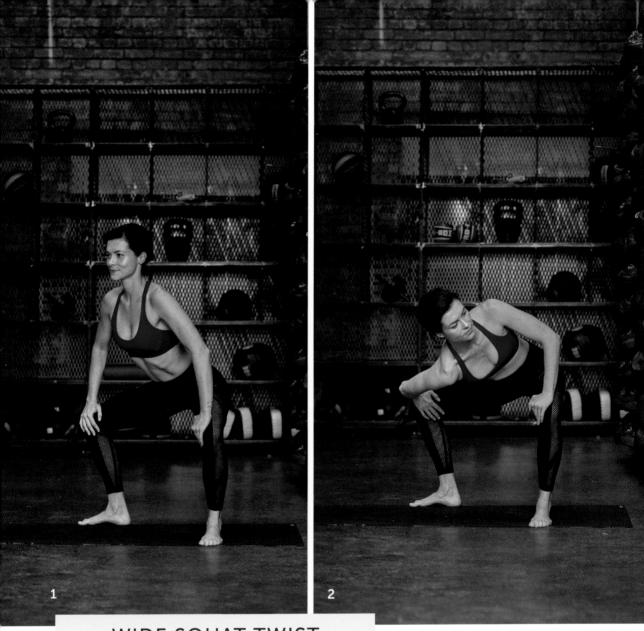

WIDE SQUAT TWIST

HOW TO DO IT: Start in a wide squat with toes pointing out. Place your hands on the insides of your knees, gently pushing outwards. Drop your left shoulder down and forwards, twisting towards your right leg. In a fluid motion, move freely from one side to the other. **{10 reps total}**

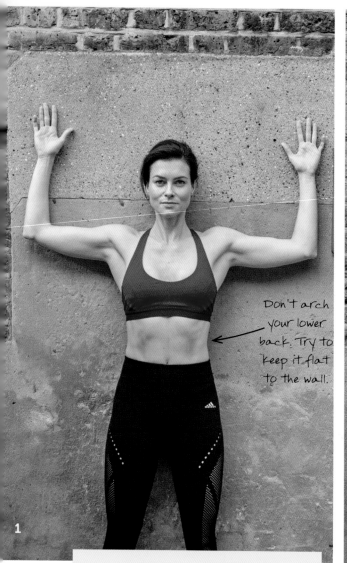

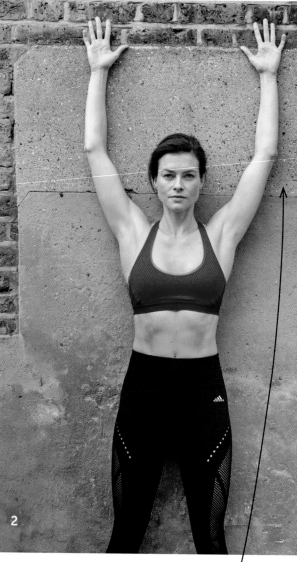

Don't arch your lower back. Try to keep it flat to the wall.

Try to keep your elbows and wrists touching the wall at all times.

WALL ANGELS

HOW TO DO IT: Stand tall, feet hip-width apart with your back to a wall (your heels a few inches away from the wall). Bend your arms at right angles and place your wrists close to the wall. Engage your core.

Straighten your arms, keeping them close to the wall. Then return to the starting position. **{10 reps}**

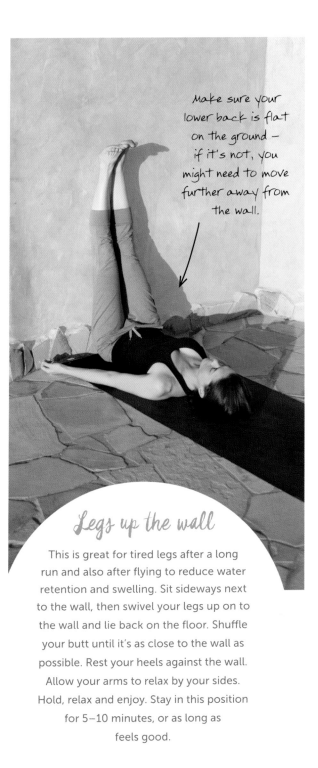

Make sure your lower back is flat on the ground — if it's not, you might need to move further away from the wall.

Legs up the wall

This is great for tired legs after a long run and also after flying to reduce water retention and swelling. Sit sideways next to the wall, then swivel your legs up on to the wall and lie back on the floor. Shuffle your butt until it's as close to the wall as possible. Rest your heels against the wall. Allow your arms to relax by your sides. Hold, relax and enjoy. Stay in this position for 5–10 minutes, or as long as feels good.

A word on posture

Sitting down for long periods, at a desk or in a car, is one of the unhealthiest things we do. The way most of us live our lives means that we're not moving our bodies as efficiently as we should, and therefore they become old and creaky before their time. However, one of the simplest ways to remedy this is to improve our posture. When we become out of alignment, due to staying hunched over in the same position for long periods, our muscles become tight and weak, which can quickly lead to lower-back and shoulder pain. We then move less, because we feel achy and stiff, and the cycle continues.

The good news is that, even if you work a 9–5 office job or sit for long periods in cars or on trains as part of your working life, you can build in some posture-perfecting stretches to your day. You can do them at your desk or at home, whenever you feel a bit 'creaky'. If I've been in the car for a long journey I'll often do a quick stretch when I get home just to 'reset' my posture and give my joints and muscles a quick straighten out.

Having little stretches throughout the day can improve your flexibility, and reduce stress and pain, so start doing these moves any time you're feeling the discomfort of being locked in one position for too long. Also try to fit in a few just before bed. The important thing to remember is to breathe normally during your stretches and only go as far as feels comfortable.

I'VE GOT YOUR BACK...
(AND NECK AND SHOULDERS)

SEATED POSTURE EXERCISES

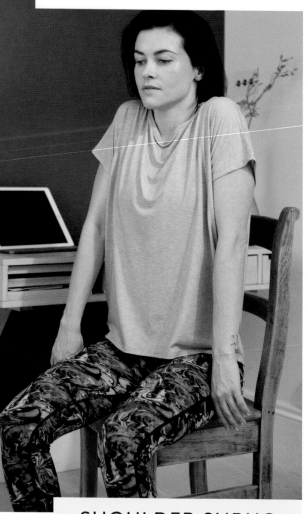

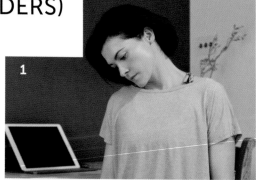

1

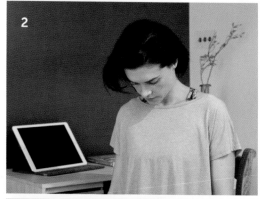

2

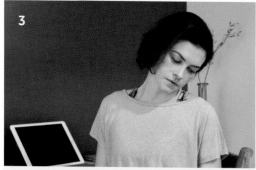

3

SHOULDER SHRUG

HOW TO DO IT: Raise both shoulders up at once towards your ears, then drop them down. **{10 reps}**

NECK STRETCH

HOW TO DO IT: Relax and lean your head forwards. Slowly roll the head to one side and hold for 10 seconds, then return to the centre and roll the head to the other side. Hold for 10 seconds. **{3 reps}**

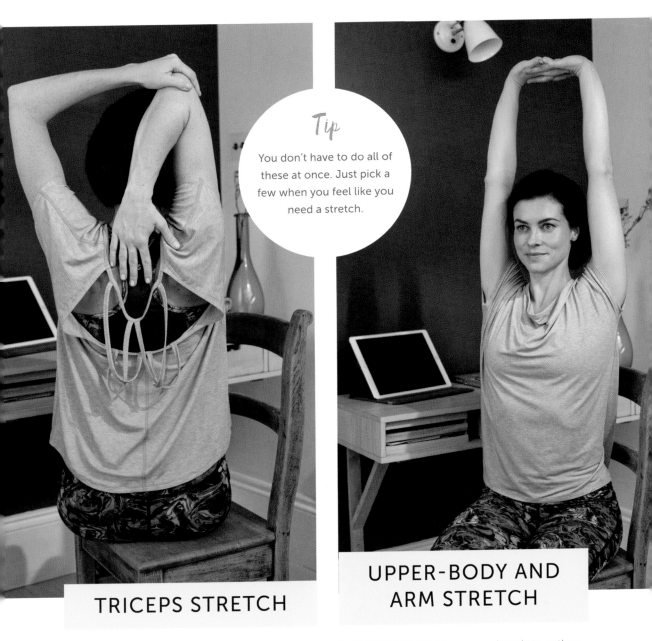

Tip

You don't have to do all of these at once. Just pick a few when you feel like you need a stretch.

TRICEPS STRETCH

UPPER-BODY AND ARM STRETCH

HOW TO DO IT: Raise one arm straight up above your head. Bend the arm at the elbow and drop the hand down. Raise your other arm and use the hand to gently pull the elbow towards the head. Hold for 10–30 seconds, then repeat on the other side.

HOW TO DO IT: Clasp your hands together above your head, palms facing outwards. Push your arms up, stretching upwards, and hold the pose for 10–30 seconds.

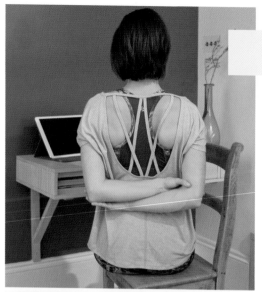

SHOULDER STRETCH

HOW TO DO IT: Cross your arms behind your back, holding on to opposite elbows and drawing the shoulder blades together. Hold the pose for 10–30 seconds.

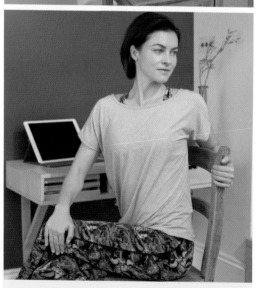

TORSO STRETCH

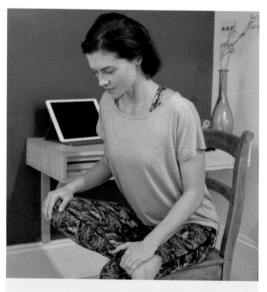

FIGURE 4

HOW TO DO IT: Cross your legs with the left leg on top. Place your right hand on your left knee and your left arm on the back of your chair, twisting your upper body to the left. Hold the pose for 10–30 seconds, then repeat on other side.

HOW TO DO IT: Sit with your left foot flat on the floor and your right ankle on your left knee, gently pressing down on the bent knee with your right hand. To increase the stretch, lean forwards a little, keeping a straight spine. Hold for 10–30 seconds. Repeat on the other side.

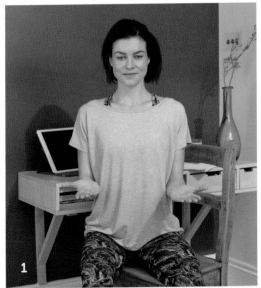

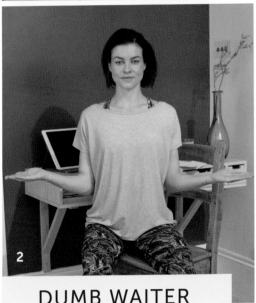

DUMB WAITER

OTHER TIPS FOR POSTURE AT WORK:

- Speak to your HR department and ask for a desk assessment to make sure your desk, chair and computer are in the best possible position for your posture.
- Walk and stand as often as possible. If you're on the phone, walk around while you chat.
- Limit time spent looking at your mobile. We all do it – whole evenings spent slouched on the sofa staring at our phones while we browse Instagram or similar. The fixed pose and repetitive movements (like swiping) can cause poor posture and pain.
- If you work in an office, always get out for a walk at lunchtime, and take small walks throughout the day if you can – go over to a colleague's desk to ask them something rather than sending an email.

HOW TO DO IT: Sit tall with both feet flat on the floor. Keeping your elbows against your side, turn your palms up as if you're holding a tray and move your hands outwards, squeezing your shoulder blades together as you do so. Return to the starting position. **{10 reps}**

COOLING DOWN

When you exercise, your muscles tear and tighten. Stretching afterwards helps bring them back to their pre-exercise state, which can reduce risk of injury, soreness and improve or maintain good mobility in the body. You must hold a stretch for at least 30 seconds in order for it to take effect, so don't rush through these. Your stretches are just as important as your main workout – don't be tempted to skip them.

- - - - - - - - - - - - - -
6 minute stretch

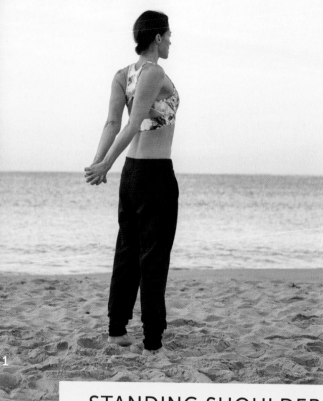

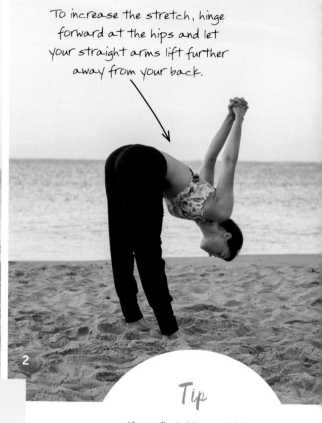

To increase the stretch, hinge forward at the hips and let your straight arms lift further away from your back.

STANDING SHOULDER STRETCH

Tip

If you find this one tricky or you have especially tight shoulders, replace it with the Shoulder stretch on page 38.

HOW TO DO IT: Stand tall and clasp your hands together behind your lower back. Keeping your arms straight, lift them away from your lower back. **{30 seconds}**

ACTIVE

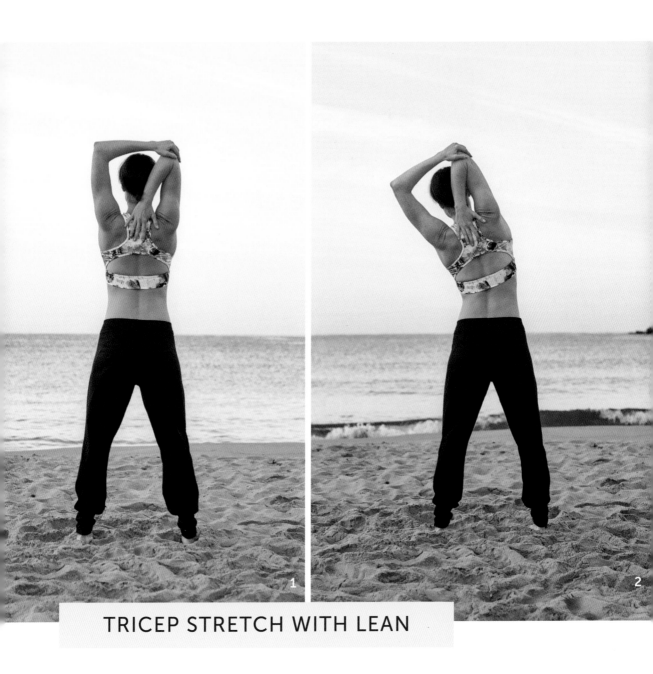

TRICEP STRETCH WITH LEAN

HOW TO DO IT: Stand tall, core engaged, with feet hip-width apart. Reach one arm straight up to the sky. Bend the elbow and drop the hand onto the top of your spine. Raise the other hand over the head and gently pull on the elbow. To increase the stretch, allow the slight pull on the elbow to cause the upper torso to lean. Repeat on the other side. **{30 seconds each side}**

LYING HAMSTRING STRETCH

HOW TO DO IT: Lie on your back with your legs straight. Bend your right knee in towards your chest, placing your hands behind your thigh. Straighten your leg up towards the sky, feeling the stretch in your hamstring. Lower and repeat with the other leg. **{30 seconds each side}**

Tip

Flex your feet to feel a greater stretch in your hamstring and calf.

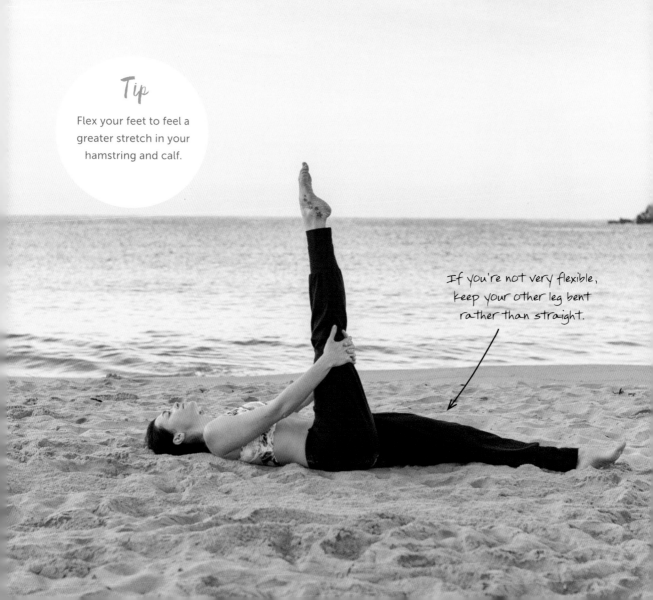

If you're not very flexible, keep your other leg bent rather than straight.

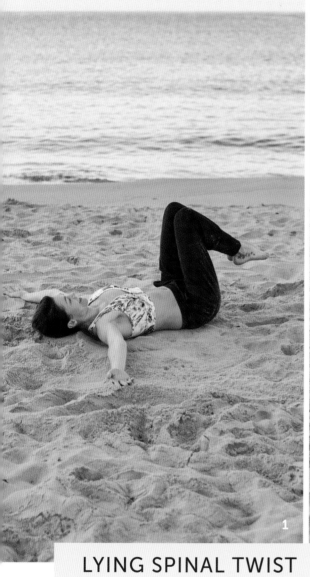

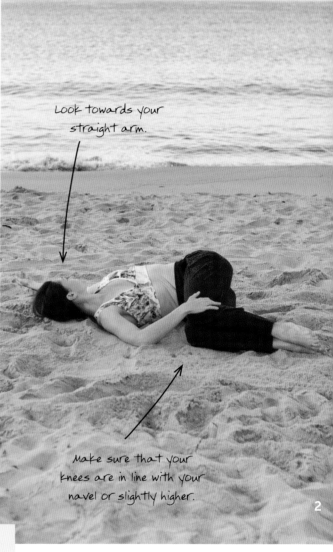

Look towards your straight arm.

Make sure that your knees are in line with your navel or slightly higher.

1

2

LYING SPINAL TWIST

HOW TO DO IT: Lie on your back with both arms stretched out at shoulder height. Bend your knees and bring them into your chest.

Keeping the knees squeezed together, let them drop to one side of your body. Use the hand closest to your knees to gently pull them to the floor. Keep your opposite shoulder and arm pinned to the floor. Repeat on the other side. **{30 seconds each side}**

Tip

As you lower your upper body, place some support under your left buttock if you need to, to keep your hips level.

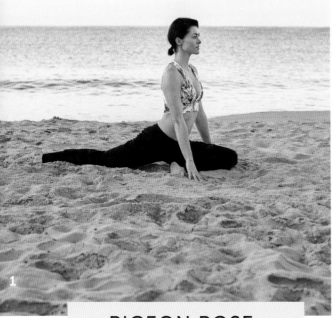

1

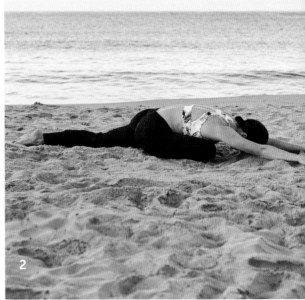

2

PIGEON POSE

HOW TO DO IT: Start on on all fours.

Slide your right shin forwards with the knee towards the right wrist, and your right ankle towards your left wrist. Slide the left leg back so it is directly behind your body.

Keeping your hands shoulder-width apart, gently lower yourself down, walking your hands forwards on the fingertips as far as you can. If it's comfortable, you can rest your forearms and forehead on the floor. Repeat on the other side. **{30 seconds each side}**

Tip

Move slowly and
smoothly from
one position to
the next.

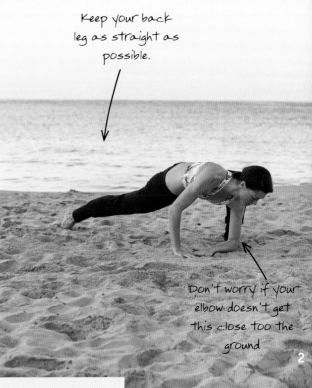

Keep your back
leg as straight as
possible.

Don't worry if your
elbow doesn't get
this close too the
ground

2

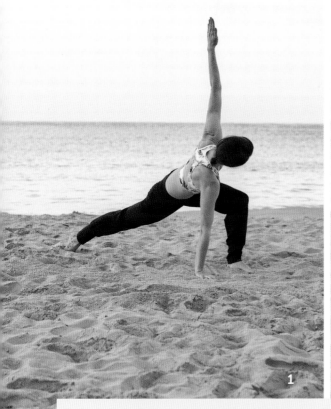

1

WORLD'S GREATEST STRETCH

HOW TO DO IT: Start in a plank position and take a big step forward with your left leg, placing your left foot to the outside of your left hand. Rotate your torso towards your bent knee and reach the left hand up to the sky.

Drop the left elbow towards the instep of your lunging foot and hold for 2 seconds. Repeat by reaching back up to the sky. Keep repeating for 30 seconds and then swap sides.
{30 seconds each side}

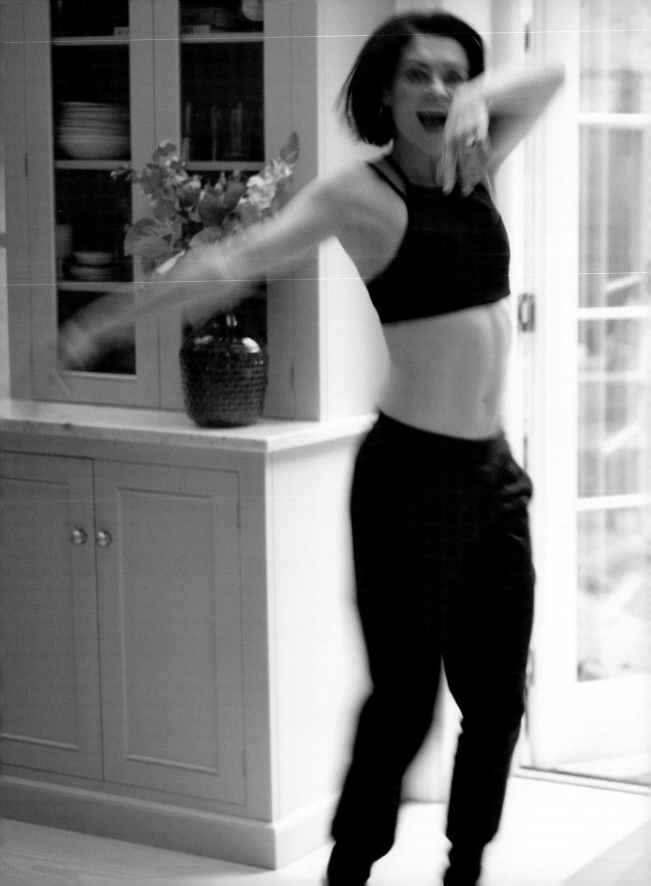

CHAPTER 2

At Home

Let's face it, your home can be a tricky place to work out. There are lots of distractions and it's very easy to be lured to the fridge or the TV, or to feel you must take care of piles of laundry. But if you can overcome this, it is the ultimate convenient location and needs no travel, no car keys, no umbrella, no nothing – you can just get on and do it.

Home workouts are also really good for mums who have young children and so can't get to the gym. The children often get involved too – and don't forget, every time you lift them up it's like lifting weights in the gym! Working out at home is also excellent for people who feel self-conscious in gyms or who don't have enough money to join one, or really don't have a lot of time and just want to squeeze in 'fitness snacks' for ten minutes at a time during a busy day.

I'll often have my best workouts at home, especially during the winter months when it can be harder to motivate myself. Often, I don't want to go out for a run in the rain or the dark but, rather than using this as an excuse for not doing anything, I see it as a time to change and adapt how I work out. Sometimes I'll just put on three or four brilliant tracks and dance around my living room, getting a sweat on for ten minutes before I jump in the shower!

HOME COMFORTS

Like I said earlier, when you're spending time at home, the kitchen can often be a scene of temptation. It's so easy, when you're stressed or bored or tired, to reach for a snack or a little pick-me-up. Therefore, when I meet new clients, I always tell them to take a look in their cupboards and fridge and assess what's there. I give them a list of items that are getting in the way of all their attempts to live a healthy lifestyle and these I tell them to clear out and throw away. Then I give them a list of items that I always keep in my kitchen and which I find help me every day to stick to my principles and enjoy fresh, healthy food.

THE 6 THINGS TO CLEAR OUT OF YOUR CUPBOARDS

- Ketchup and sauces – they're full of hidden sugar. If you cook with fresh, flavoursome ingredients and season with herbs and spices, you don't need to add sugary, processed flavours.
- Cereals – again, they're packed with hidden sugar. Turn to pages 145–51 instead for some breakfast ideas.
- Ready-made meals for the freezer – these are packed with salt, sugar and processed additives and are less nutritious than home-prepared foods. Avoid! Make your own meals and freeze those instead.
- Treats – So many people keep a 'naughty drawer' full of sugary sweets and treats, but I tell my clients that if it's in your house, you'll eat it, especially when you're at a low ebb. So don't buy biscuits and ice cream out of habit because you'll eat them out of habit too.
- Sugary drinks/fizzy sodas – again, these are packed with sugar. Stick to water or herbal teas instead (page 162 for infused waters).
- Low-fat anything – many studies now prove what a lot of health experts have been saying for years. Low-fat foods, like 'diet' yogurts, drinks, ready meals and so on, are often packed with processed sweeteners that can disrupt your metabolism and make you hungrier and more likely to gain and hold onto excess weight.

THE 6 THINGS TO KEEP IN YOUR CUPBOARDS

- Always have chopped-up raw veg (carrots, sweet peppers, cucumbers, celery) ready in the fridge for easy snacks.
- Almond butter – great for a quick snack spread on a buckwheat cracker or a slice of apple.
- A homemade, healthy frozen meal for emergencies.
- Eggs! Healthy, delicious and easy for breakfast, lunch or dinner. Omelette, scrambled eggs, frittata... eggs are so versatile and full of protein.
- Dark chocolate – we all have moments of craving. A small amount of dark chocolate can satisfy that desire without feeding the sugar addiction.
- Seeds and nuts – great for a quick snack.

MY 6 TOP KITCHEN ITEMS

- Vitamix – I use this to make everything from my morning smoothies, to soups, dips, sauces and energy balls (pages 145–67 for my recipes).
- A vegetable peeler – a simple potato peeler can double up as a spiraliser and be used to turn raw vegetables like carrots and courgettes into ribbons.
- Glass Tupperware – I'm a bit picky about Tupperware and I don't really like using plastic. If I do use plastic, it has to be BPA-free. But mostly I use glass Tupperware. It's great for batch cooking and storing homemade meals that I can heat up quickly when I get home from work late or if I'm going out for the day and won't have access to anything healthy.
- BPA-free water bottle – you can buy the ones with a funnel through the middle where you can put in fruits, vegetables or herbs to flavour the water. Or you can just add these natural flavourings to a regular water bottle like this.
- Coffee machine – if you're a coffee fan, invest in a good machine. It's really worth it – I buy freshly ground organic coffee beans, which taste amazing. Just think about this for a moment – if you get a take away coffee three times a week, that's 156 times a year. If you spend £3 each time, that comes to £468 annually. That could be going towards a gym membership, new workout gear... or a holiday!

ANNELISE, 42, IT SPECIALIST AND MUM OF TWO

'In recent years, my marriage ended and I became a single parent. I went from having my husband at home, which gave me the flexibility to go to the gym at the weekend or after work, to trying to find new ways to fit exercise into my new life. It was hard. I couldn't find a way to make it work and yet I needed to because by then exercise had become my salvation. So Holly started training me at home, with my children watching and sometimes even joining in!

'So now I find ways to involve my kids in what I do. As well as working out at home, I might run along behind my kids when they go out for a bike ride. If we're on holiday, I'll swim in the sea while they're on a surfboard or dingy, paddling along beside me – and we all take turns on the trampoline in the garden.

'I genuinely feel like I'm a better mum when I exercise. I find it so empowering and my newfound fitness gives me so much pride. I can run to catch a bus and do cartwheels on the beach with the kids. I also love showing my children what exercise is. Even if that's getting them to time me while I do a plank (they always laugh at me while I'm doing it!), having handstand competitions or taking part in fun runs together. So many mums get this martyr addiction, where they do everything for everybody else. But you need to look after yourself first in order to look after others.'

GET LIVELY IN THE LIVING ROOM

This workout is contained to a small area, so even if you don't have a huge amount of space in your living room, you can do this. It's a full-body work-out based around your sofa – you can even do it while you're watching TV! Most of the exercises in this book can be done without any equipment. However, there are a few things I suggest my clients buy to add a bit of variety to their workouts, including loop bands, which are used in this workout. They add resistance to your workouts and can be used for stretching and to help with posture. They are inexpensive, versatile and can be taken anywhere (i.e. on holiday with you). If you don't have any, don't worry – you can still do these exercises without them. Remember to warm up first (pages 22–38). Repeat this whole workout three times

- - - - - - - - - - - - - - -

**12 minute workout
(3 x 4 minutes)**

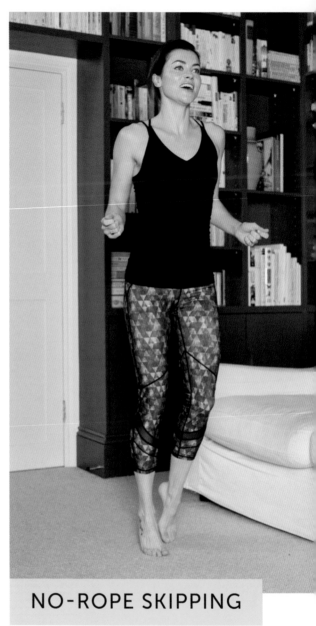

Circuits

Every workout in this book is in a circuit style, which means you do each exercise one after the other, then go back to the beginning of the circuit and repeat.

NO-ROPE SKIPPING

HOW TO DO IT: Simply pretend you have a rope in your hands and skip for 30 seconds.
{30 seconds}

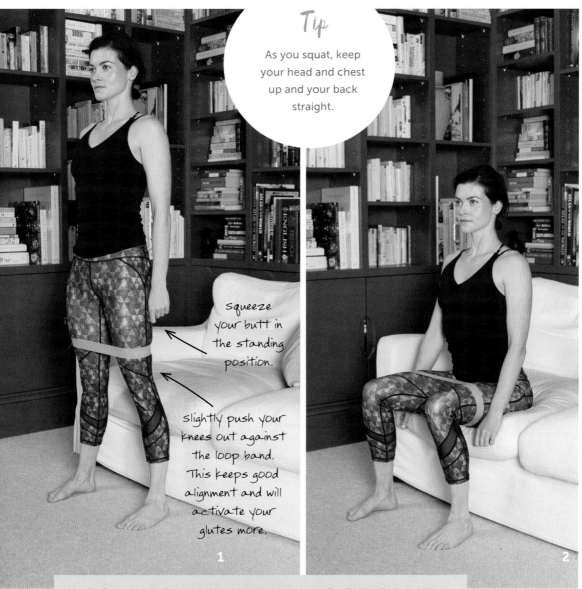

Tip

As you squat, keep your head and chest up and your back straight.

Squeeze your butt in the standing position.

Slightly push your knees out against the loop band. This keeps good alignment and will activate your glutes more.

1

2

SOFA SQUAT WITH A LOOP BAND

HOW TO DO IT: Place a loop band around both legs, just above the knees. Stand up straight in front of the sofa with your core engaged and feet shoulder-width apart.

Squat down, lowering your butt towards the sofa and sit down – but don't stop there!
Keeping the weight in your heels, push back up to standing. **{10 reps}**

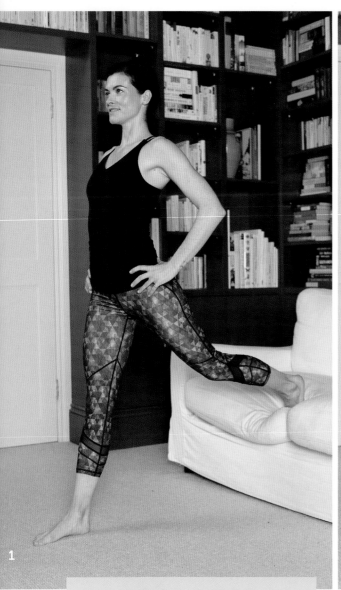

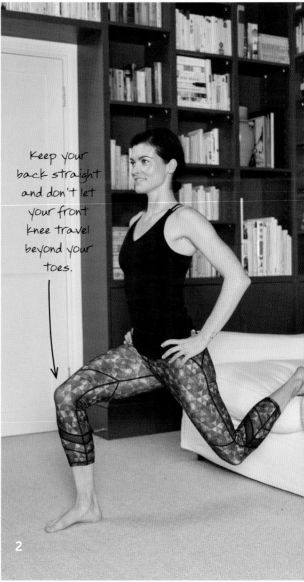

Keep your back straight and don't let your front knee travel beyond your toes.

1

2

SOFA LUNGE

HOW TO DO IT: Stand about two feet away from the sofa. Lift one leg and place the foot on the sofa behind you.

Bend both knees until your front thigh is almost horizontal. Hold for a moment, then push up through your front heel and return to the start position. **{10 reps each side}**

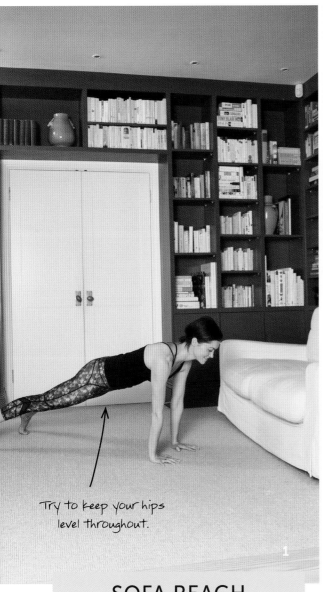

Try to keep your hips level throughout.

1

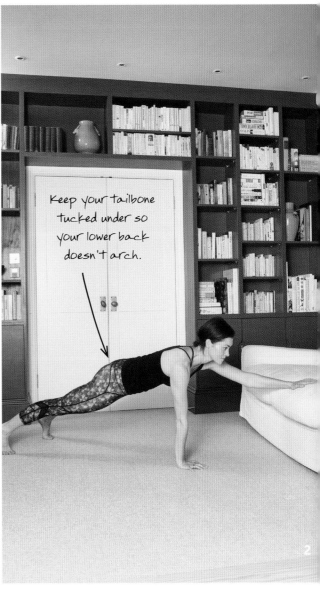

Keep your tailbone tucked under so your lower back doesn't arch.

2

SOFA REACH

HOW TO DO IT: Start in a high plank position with your body in a straight line from the head to the heels, about an arm's length away from the sofa. Engage your core.

Lift one hand and reach it out in front of you to touch the sofa. Hold for a moment. Return your hand to the floor and repeat the movement with the other hand. **{10 reps total}**

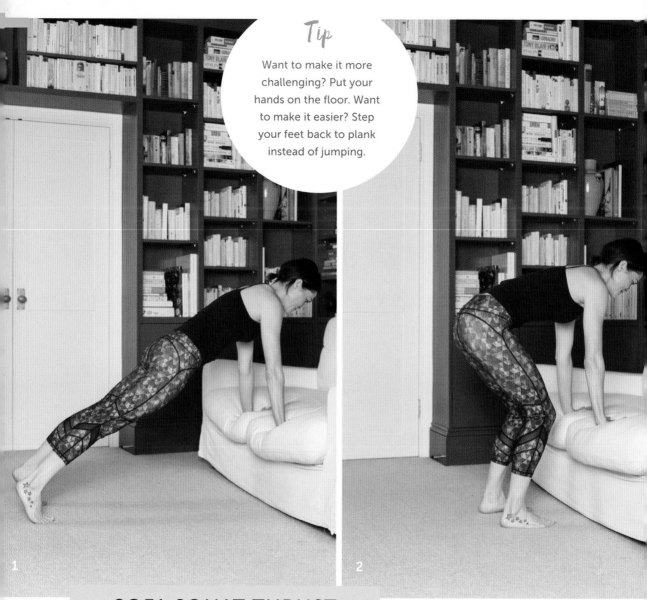

Tip

Want to make it more challenging? Put your hands on the floor. Want to make it easier? Step your feet back to plank instead of jumping.

1

2

SOFA SQUAT THRUST

HOW TO DO IT: Start in a high plank position with your hands on the edge of the sofa and your body in a straight line from the head to the heels.

Jump both feet towards your hands, landing with them hip-width apart.

Explosively kick both feet back into the plank position. Keep jumping back and forth.

{20 reps}

SOFA GLUTE BRIDGE

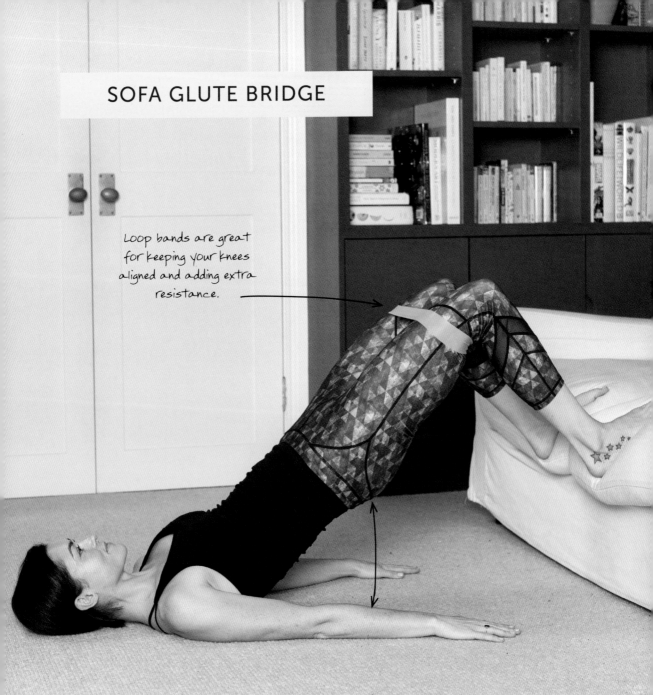

Loop bands are great for keeping your knees aligned and adding extra resistance.

HOW TO DO IT: Place a loop band around your legs, just above the knees, and lie back on the floor. Lift your legs and place both feet, hip-distance apart, on the edge of the sofa. Squeeze your glutes and push your hips off the floor until your knees, hips and shoulders are all in a straight line. Hold for a moment, then lower back down. **{10 reps}**

QUICK KITCHEN WORKOUT

You don't have to get your heart racing to have a good workout. Here's one that will tone and sculpt – a full-body workout, without the cardio element. It means you might not even break a sweat – perfect if you're just waiting for the dinner to cook and don't want to have to take a shower afterwards. All you need is a tea towel – your kitchen doesn't just have to be a place for putting on the pounds! Remember to warm up first (pages 22–38) Repeat each exercise in this workout for 30 seconds at a time, and repeat the whole workout three times.

- -
15 minutes (3 x 5 minutes)

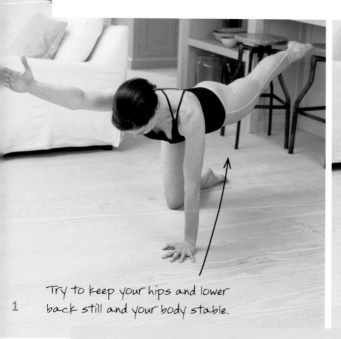

1   Try to keep your hips and lower back still and your body stable.

2   Inhale as you reach out, exhale as you draw in.

BIRD-DOG

HOW TO DO IT: Start on all fours. Without allowing your lower back to rise or round, draw your belly in and engage your core.

Raise your right arm and left leg until they are in line with your body. Pause for a second then draw the arm and leg in under the body so the hand touches the knee. Keep repeating the movement for 30 seconds, then change to the other side. **{30 seconds each side}**

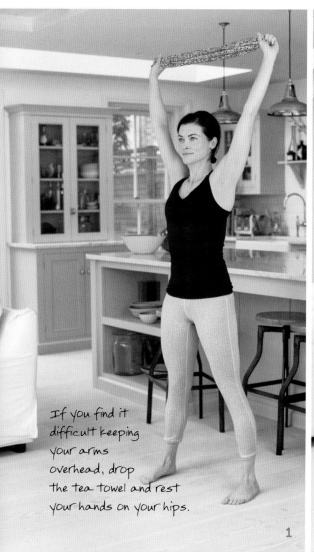

Tip

This is great for undoing some of the damage that prolonged sitting can do to the body as it opens up hamstring flexibility and hip-joint mobility.

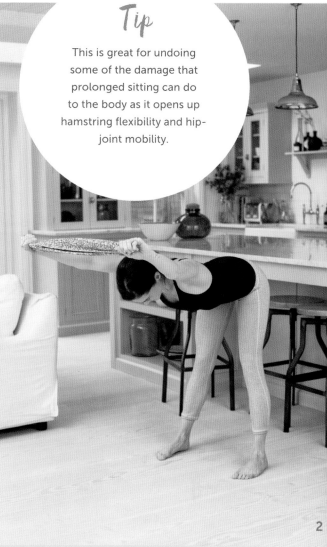

If you find it difficult keeping your arms overhead, drop the tea towel and rest your hands on your hips.

1

2

HIP-HINGE WITH TEA TOWEL REACH

HOW TO DO IT: Stand tall with your feet slightly wider than hip-distance apart and hold a tea towel above your head.

Hinge forwards at the hips, keeping your spine straight (don't round it). Imagine there is a wall behind you and you are trying to tap your butt against it. Pause, then return to the start position, keeping your arms in line with your ears. **{30 seconds total}**

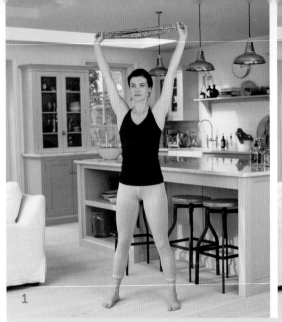
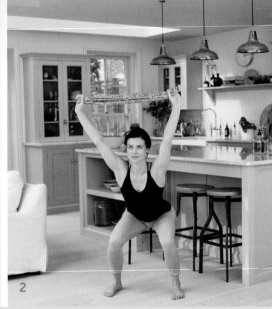

OVERHEAD WIDE SQUAT WITH SIDE BENDS

Tip

You want the tea towel to be tight, so keep your arms and upper back strong and your core engaged.

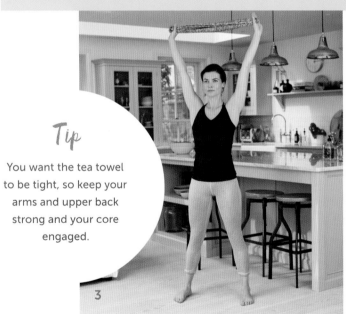
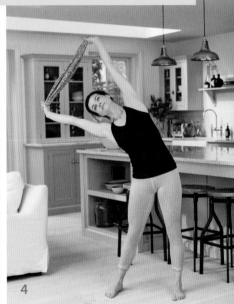

HOW TO DO IT: Stand tall with your feet slightly wider than hip-distance apart and hold a tea towel above your head.

Slowly bend your knees into a squat, keeping your chest lifted and your arms straight. Pause, then return to standing.

With your arms and upper back still strong and straight, bend to the right side, then return to the centre and bend to the left side. Return to the start position.

{30 seconds total}

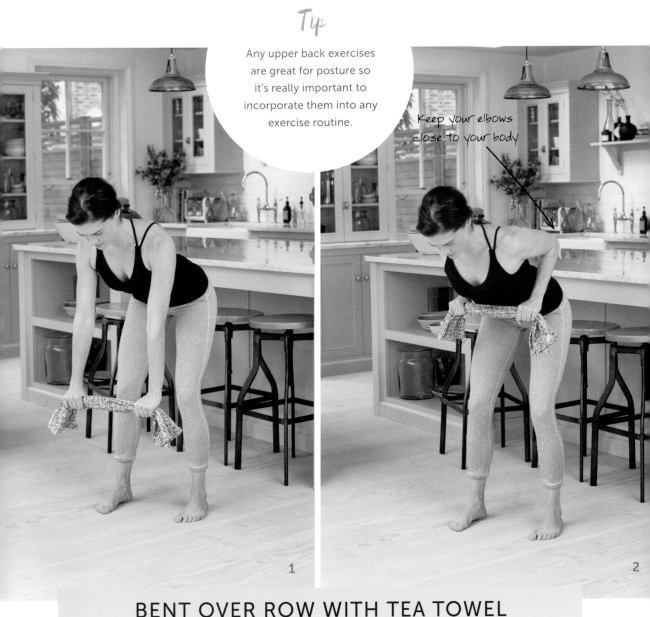

Tip

Any upper back exercises are great for posture so it's really important to incorporate them into any exercise routine.

Keep your elbows close to your body

1

2

BENT OVER ROW WITH TEA TOWEL

HOW TO DO IT: Start with your feet hip-width apart, holding a tea towel as shown. Slightly bend your knees, hinge forwards at the hips and let the arms hang. Pull the tea towel up to your chest and squeeze your shoulder blades together while drawing down your back in a rowing motion. Pause, then straighten the arms. **{30 seconds total}**

BACK EXTENSION WITH REACH

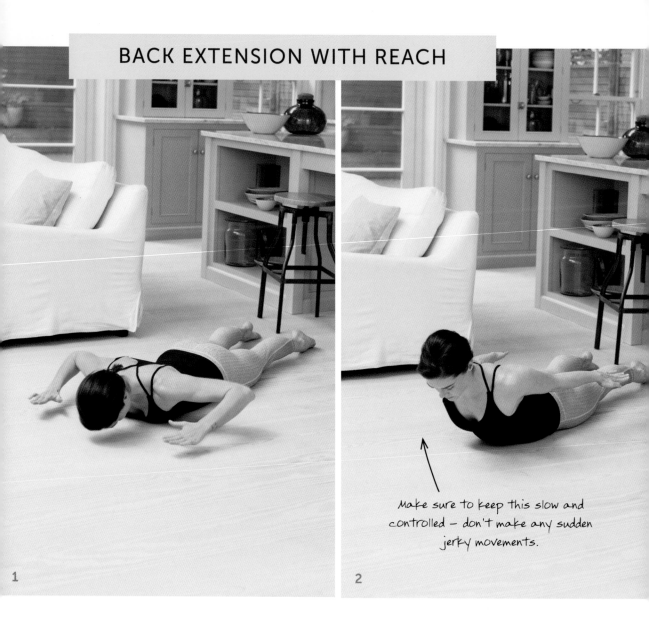

Make sure to keep this slow and controlled — don't make any sudden jerky movements.

1

2

HOW TO DO IT: Start lying face-down on the floor, with both legs extended out straight, and your elbows at right angles.

Extend your spine and lift your chest and arms off the ground. Draw the elbows back, straighten your arms and reach back towards your feet. Hold, then slowly lower yourself back to the floor, bringing your arms back to right angles. **{30 seconds total}**

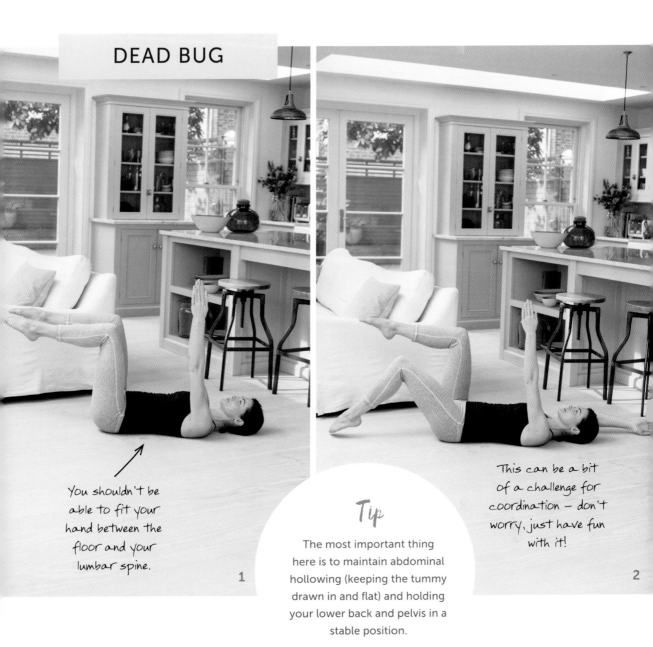

DEAD BUG

You shouldn't be able to fit your hand between the floor and your lumbar spine.

1

Tip

The most important thing here is to maintain abdominal hollowing (keeping the tummy drawn in and flat) and holding your lower back and pelvis in a stable position.

This can be a bit of a challenge for coordination — don't worry, just have fun with it!

2

HOW TO DO IT: Lie flat on your back with your arms extended above you towards the ceiling. Bend your legs and lift so your knees are aligned with your hips and your shins are parallel to the floor. Engage your core to bring your ribcage down and flatten your back to the floor.

Slowly lower the right arm behind your head and the left leg down to the floor. Slowly return to the starting position. Repeat with the opposite arm and leg. **{30 seconds total}**

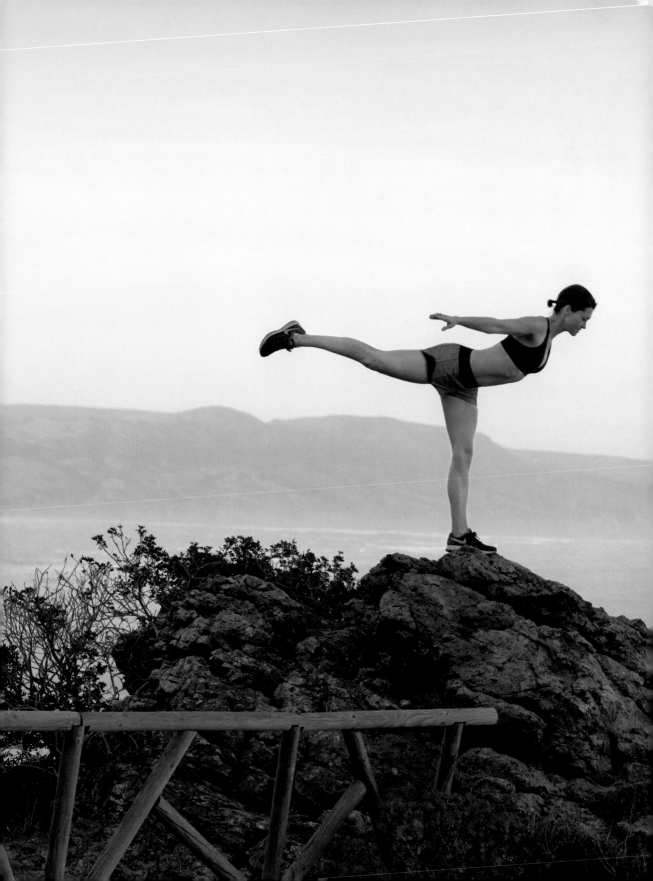

CHAPTER 3

Take it Outside

I've always loved exercising outside and often run round my local streets and take my workouts to the park. Being in the fresh air and having a connection with nature – whether it's drizzling rain or bright sunshine – always melts away my stress and I come home feeling energised and happy. I live in a busy part of London, but I can always find a green, hilly or open space to run around in, or take a brisk walk through. I'll use benches in my local park for press-ups or triceps-dips.

I often ask my clients why they enjoy exercising outside and they say that they love the fact it's always different – the views, the seasons, the sounds. It's invigorating and also makes them feel calmer. And it seems we may be on to something. Researchers from the University of Innsbruck in Austria have found that the mood-improving and anxiety-reducing benefits of exercise are greater when that exercise happens outside rather than in a gym. So I'll always encourage my clients to do at least one of their workouts outside. Wherever you live, try to make the most of the great outdoors and all the free health benefits that it offers.

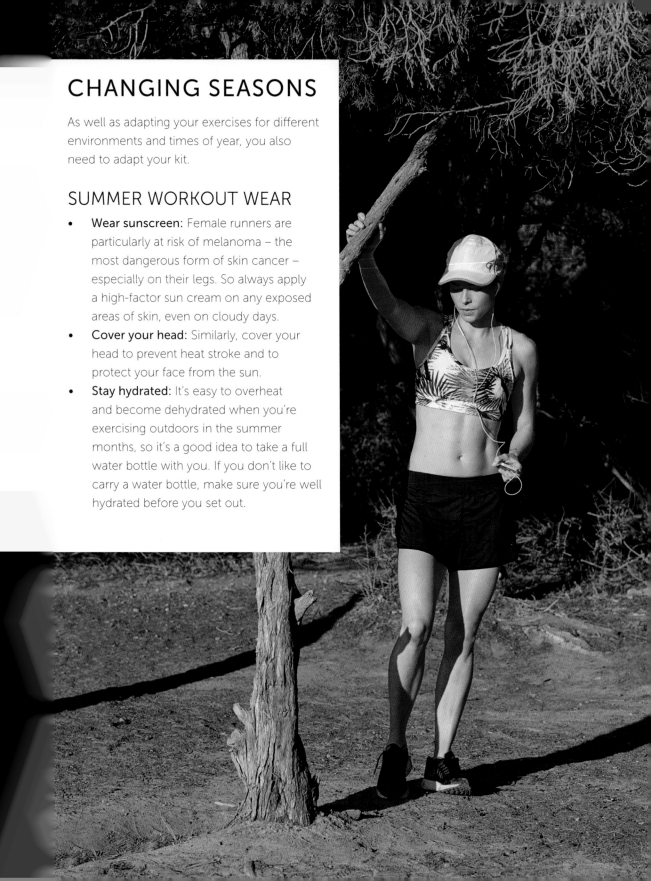

CHANGING SEASONS

As well as adapting your exercises for different environments and times of year, you also need to adapt your kit.

SUMMER WORKOUT WEAR

- **Wear sunscreen:** Female runners are particularly at risk of melanoma – the most dangerous form of skin cancer – especially on their legs. So always apply a high-factor sun cream on any exposed areas of skin, even on cloudy days.
- **Cover your head:** Similarly, cover your head to prevent heat stroke and to protect your face from the sun.
- **Stay hydrated:** It's easy to overheat and become dehydrated when you're exercising outdoors in the summer months, so it's a good idea to take a full water bottle with you. If you don't like to carry a water bottle, make sure you're well hydrated before you set out.

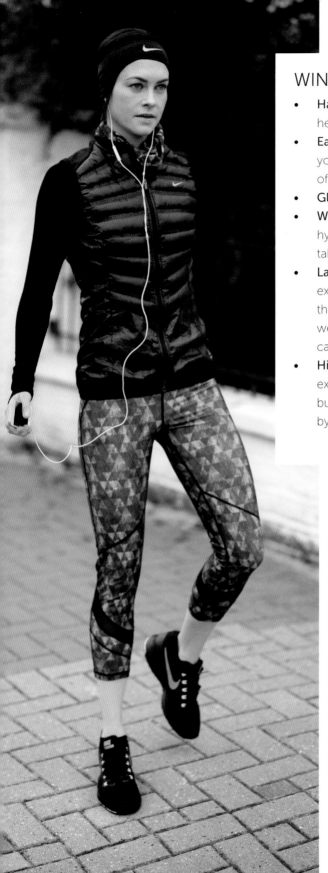

WINTER WORKOUT WEAR

- **Hat:** We lose a lot of our body heat through our heads so, on particularly cold days, wear a hat.
- **Ear muffs or a head band:** Cold ears may cause you to cut your run short, so get yourself a pair of earmuffs.
- **Gloves or long sleeves:** Ditto icy fingers.
- **Water:** Even on cold days you need to stay hydrated, so either drink water before you go or take a water bottle with you.
- **Layers:** Wear a few thin layers when you're exercising outside in winter, so you can peel them off as you become hotter, rather than wearing a big bulky running top that could cause you to overheat.
- **High vis:** This is especially important if you're exercising in the evenings and running around busy roads. You'll be more likely to be spotted by traffic and passers-by.

AMIE, 42, FASHION PR
AND MUM OF THREE

'Holly helped me find a way of fitting fitness into my busy life, juggling three children and a stressful job. Together, we looked at my life, my work, my moods and we adapted my workouts to fit around everything.

'After a stressful day, I often don't feel like doing anything too heavy and will do some yoga instead. Holly also encourages clients to change their workouts according to the seasons and I'll often think, "Right, spring is here, I'm going to run outside."

FULL-BODY BLAST

This is a high-intensity, invigorating workout. These exercises can be done outside with no equipment. Perform each one for 30 seconds and rest for 15 seconds in between (if you need it). Always warm up first (pages 22–39). One circuit should take about 6 minutes and I recommend you try to do 3 rounds. Rest and drink some water between circuits. | **18 minutes (3 x 6 minutes)**

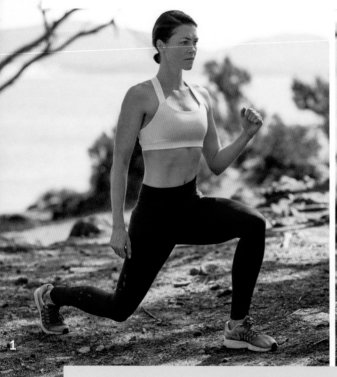

REVERSE LUNGE WITH KNEE DRIVE

HOW TO DO IT: Stand tall and take a big step back, bending both knees so your back knee nearly touches the floor. With a big push off the back foot, come up to balance on one leg with the bent knee raised to your chest and pause. Without your foot touching the floor, step straight back into the lunge. Repeat for 30 seconds, then swap sides. **{30 seconds each side}**

Tip

To make it easier, don't do the knee drive, just place your foot next to the other after the lunge. Want a challenge? Add a hop at the top.

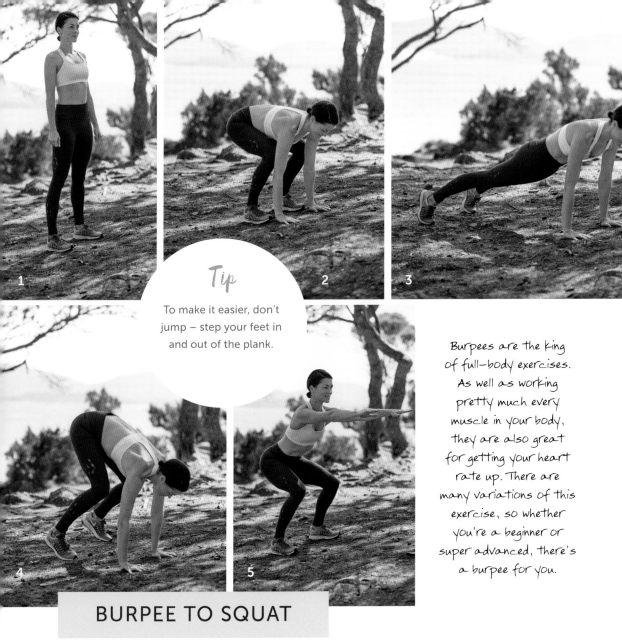

Tip

To make it easier, don't jump – step your feet in and out of the plank.

Burpees are the king of full-body exercises. As well as working pretty much every muscle in your body, they are also great for getting your heart rate up. There are many variations of this exercise, so whether you're a beginner or super advanced, there's a burpee for you.

BURPEE TO SQUAT

HOW TO DO IT: Stand tall, feet hip-width apart, then bend both knees and place your hands flat on the floor.

Keeping your core engaged, jump both feet back so you are in a high plank position.

Jump your feet forward so they land directly behind your hands. Lift your hands off the floor but keep your butt down to hold a squat. Don't come up to stand, but rather place your hands back on the floor and jump straight back into plank and your next rep. **{30 seconds total}**

SIDE LUNGE KNEE RAISE

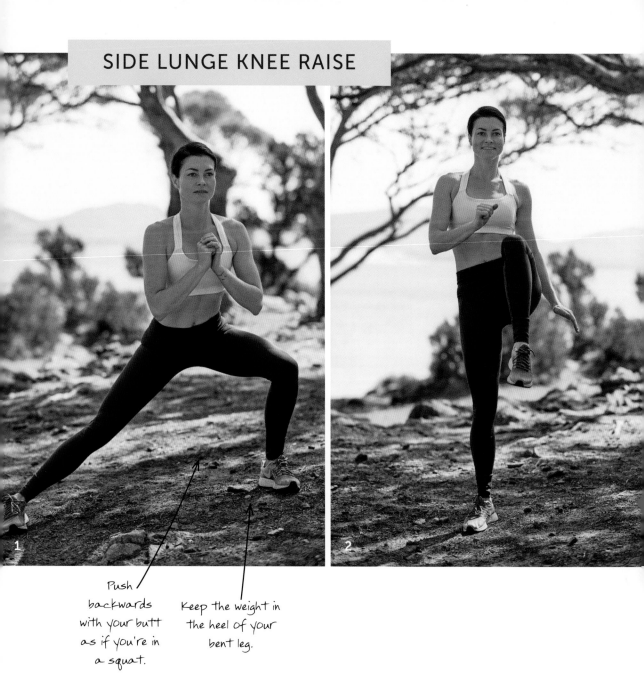

Push backwards with your butt as if you're in a squat.

Keep the weight in the heel of your bent leg.

HOW TO DO IT: Start with your feet hip-width apart. Take a big step and lunge to the left, keeping your right leg completely straight. Big push off your left foot to bring your left knee up to your chest. Go straight back into the side lunge. Repeat this movement for 30 seconds, then do the other side. **{30 seconds each side}**

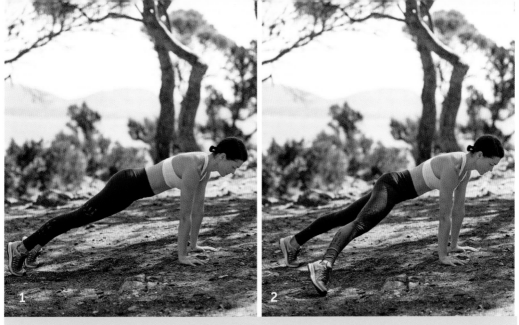

PLANK TOE TAPS TO MOUNTAIN CLIMBER

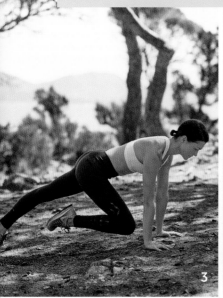

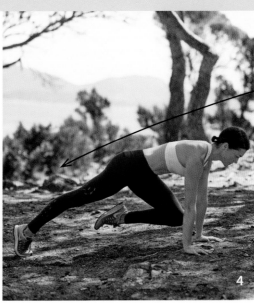

It's important to keep a straight line from your shoulders to your heels – don't let your butt lift up or your hips drop.

HOW TO DO IT: Start in a high plank position with your shoulders over your wrists and feet together.

Lift one leg out wide to the side and let your foot tap the floor, then bring it back to the start position and repeat with the other leg.

Stay in a plank position, and bring one knee up to your chest, then return the leg to the start position and repeat on the other side – this is the mountain climber. Repeat.

{30 seconds total}

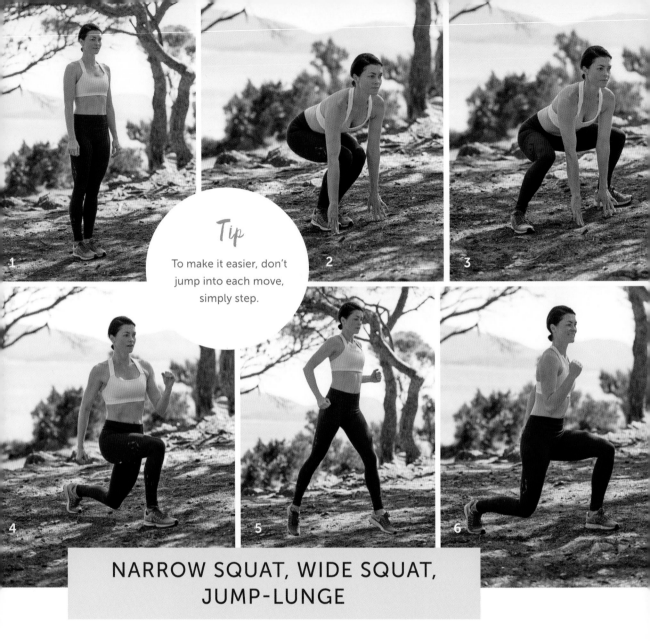

Tip

To make it easier, don't jump into each move, simply step.

NARROW SQUAT, WIDE SQUAT, JUMP-LUNGE

HOW TO DO IT: Stand tall with your core engaged and feet together, then squat down, touching the floor with your fingertips.

Staying low with your upper body, jump your feet out to a wide squat, again touching the floor. Then lift your upper body and jump into a lunge position with the right leg forwards and the left back. Jump to swap legs, bringing the left leg forwards and the right back, then jump both feet back together into the narrow squat. Repeat. **{30 seconds total}**

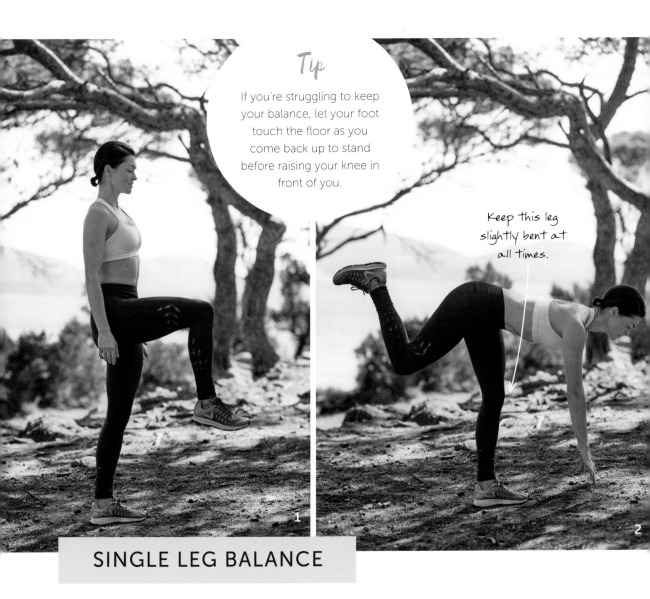

Tip

If you're struggling to keep your balance, let your foot touch the floor as you come back up to stand before raising your knee in front of you.

Keep this leg slightly bent at all times.

1

2

SINGLE LEG BALANCE

HOW TO DO IT: Stand tall with your feet shoulder-width apart, your core engaged and both knees slightly bent. Lift your right knee towards your chest. Hinge at at your hips, keep your back straight and lower your torso forwards.

Briefly pause, then return to the knee raise. Repeat for 30 seconds without your foot touching the floor, then repeat on the other side. **{30 seconds each side}**

BODY BENCH WORKOUT

A simple park bench provides the best piece of equipment for an outdoor workout and you can find them everywhere. This is a high intensity workout that uses your own body weight. Each circuit will take about 4 minutes in total. Depending on how much time you have, or how much of a challenge you want, repeat 3, 4 or 5 times.

- -

12 minutes (3 x 4 minutes)
16 minutes (4 x 4 minutes)
20 minutes (5 x 4 minutes)

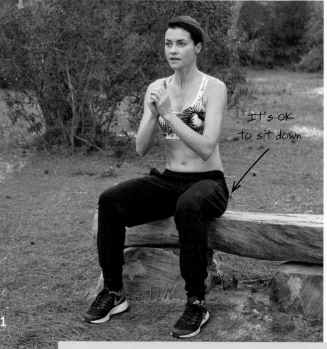

It's OK to sit down

1

2

BENCH SQUAT JUMPS

HOW TO DO IT: Stand in front of a bench with your core engaged and feet shoulder-width apart. Keeping your back straight, push your hips back and bend your knees to lower yourself onto the bench. As soon as your butt touches the bench, jump up. **{10 reps}**

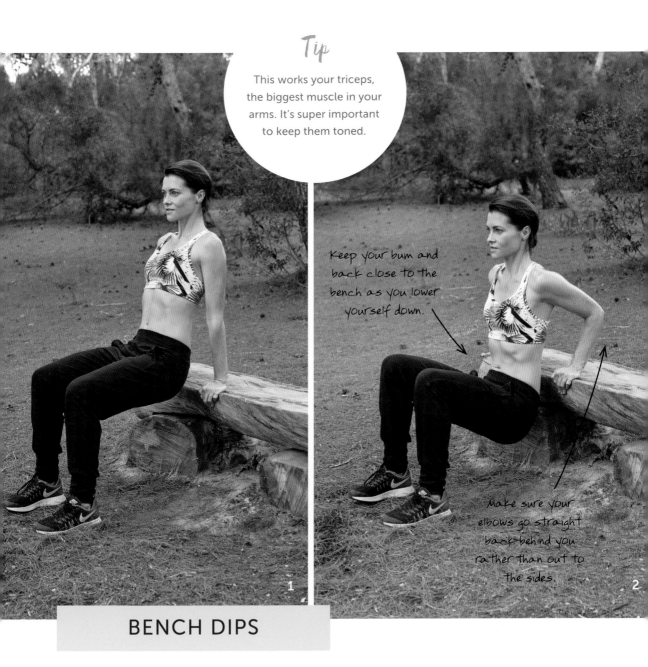

Tip

This works your triceps, the biggest muscle in your arms. It's super important to keep them toned.

Keep your bum and back close to the bench as you lower yourself down.

Make sure your elbows go straight back behind you rather than out to the sides.

1

2

BENCH DIPS

HOW TO DO IT: Sit on the edge of a bench with your hands gripping the edge of the seat. Shuffle your butt off the bench so your arms are supporting your weight and lower yourself a few inches. Pause at the bottom, then push back up to straighten your arms. **{10 reps}**

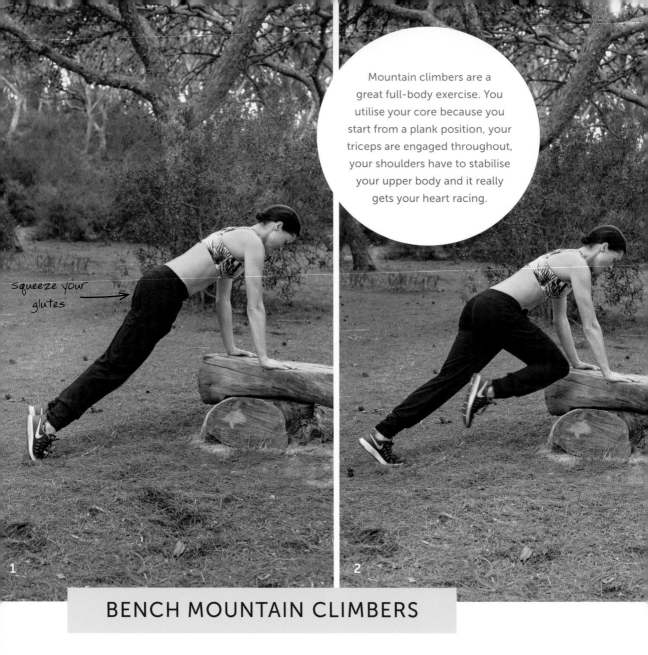

Mountain climbers are a great full-body exercise. You utilise your core because you start from a plank position, your triceps are engaged throughout, your shoulders have to stabilise your upper body and it really gets your heart racing.

squeeze your glutes →

1

2

BENCH MOUNTAIN CLIMBERS

HOW TO DO IT: Start in a high plank position with your hands on the bench. Keep your core engaged and your body in a straight line from your heels to your head.

Without lifting your butt up into the air, drive one knee into your chest.

Quickly switch legs, pulling the opposite knee in as you push your right leg back, and keep the momentum going. **{20 reps total, 10 each side.}**

ACTIVE

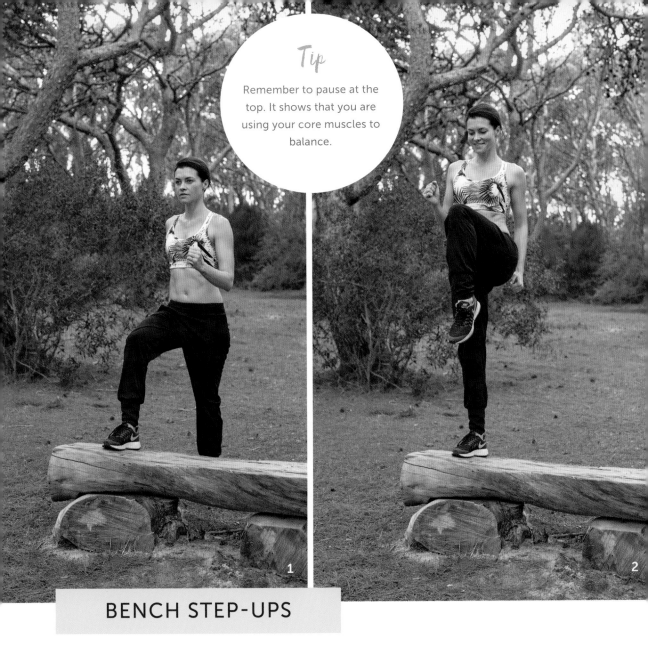

Tip

Remember to pause at the top. It shows that you are using your core muscles to balance.

1

2

BENCH STEP-UPS

HOW TO DO IT: Stand facing a bench and place your entire right foot on the bench in front of you. Press through your right heel and step up, bringing your left knee up towards your chest. Straighten your right knee to stand on the bench. Hold at the top to check good balance and core control, then return your left foot to the floor. Keep your right foot on the bench until all reps are completed, then swap legs. **{20 reps total, 10 each side.}**

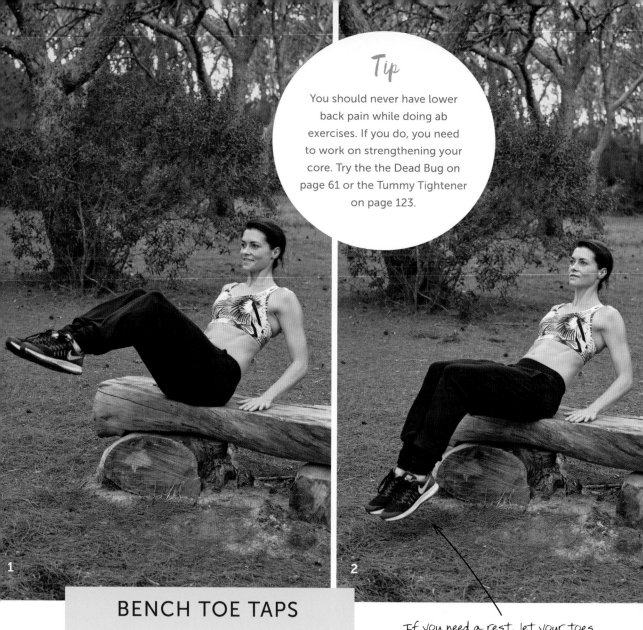

Tip

You should never have lower back pain while doing ab exercises. If you do, you need to work on strengthening your core. Try the the Dead Bug on page 61 or the Tummy Tightener on page 123.

BENCH TOE TAPS

If you need a rest, let your toes rest on the floor for a moment and then get back into it.

HOW TO DO IT: Sit on the edge of the bench with your hands resting on the bench. Keeping your spine straight, lean back a little and slightly lift your feet.

Slowly lift your knees towards your chest for a count of three, pause at the top, then slowly lower for a count of three. Don't let your toes touch the ground until you have completed 10 reps. **{10 reps}**

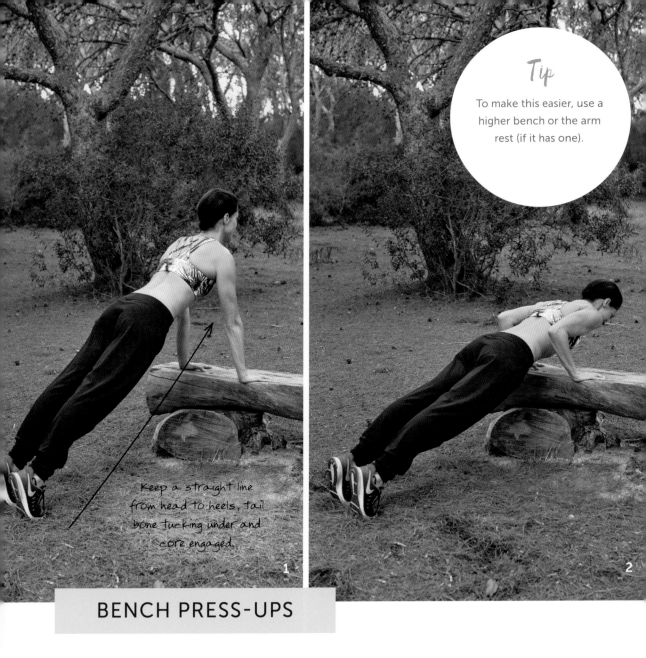

Tip

To make this easier, use a higher bench or the arm rest (if it has one).

Keep a straight line from head to heels, tail bone tucking under and core engaged.

1

2

BENCH PRESS-UPS

HOW TO DO IT: Start in a high plank position with your hands slightly wider than shoulder-width apart on the bench and your feet close together on the ground. Tucking your elbows in, lower yourself down towards the seat (with your chest as close as it can go). Pause at the bottom, before pushing your body back up to the start position. **{10 reps}**

A GUIDE TO GETTING STARTED WITH RUNNING

DON'T SET OFF TOO FAST

It sounds obvious, but we're often so eager to get started that we power off at a great speed but then find ourselves gasping for breath, heading home and feeling put off running for at least another couple of months. So take it slow and don't push yourself too hard at the start. The first few minutes of a run should be about allowing your lungs to open up and your body to warm up. Then after that, keep a steady pace that you can comfortably manage and build up your pace and distance. Sustainability is key.

PICK YOUR RUNNING BUDDY WISELY

I highly recommend running with a friend for encouragement, motivation and company. However, pick them wisely. If they're much faster than you are, you'll either set off at the wrong pace and not be able to run for as long or as far, or you'll become disheartened and are then much more likely to give up. So pick a friend who has roughly the same running ability as you and again, build up slowly.

DON'T GET TOO COMFORTABLE

Once you get going, if you find yourself having to slow to a walk to catch your breath, try and start a gentle jog (building into a slightly quicker one) again as soon as possible. It's very easy to get too comfortable in a walk.

PICK YOUR BEST ROUTE

Some people love routine and want to stick with the same route every time they run, while others need to keep mixing it up and finding new places to explore in order to keep it fresh and interesting. See what works for you. It never hurts to break out of your comfort zone a little though, and adding in a gentle hill or change of scenery can give you a little boost if you start to become bored.

TRY AN APP

Apps can be a great support and provide you with lots of info that enables you to track your progress, which can then give you an extra boost of motivation. If you really enjoy using one, think about getting a fitness tracker, like a Fitbit or Apple watch.

RUN OUTSIDE

Treadmills can be great for running, especially on those dark winter evenings when you feel like staying warm and dry. But nothing beats being outside. I always urge my clients to run outside and enjoy the fresh air and the ever-changing seasons and surroundings. No run is ever the same when you're outside. However, if you do run on a treadmill, remember to add in some inclines!

SIGN UP FOR A RACE

This provides the best running motivation ever. Start small with a 5 or 10k, do it for a charity close to your heart as this will bind you to your commitment and encourage some friends to run it with you. You'll feel such a sense of achievement crossing that finish line – you'll want to do it again and again.

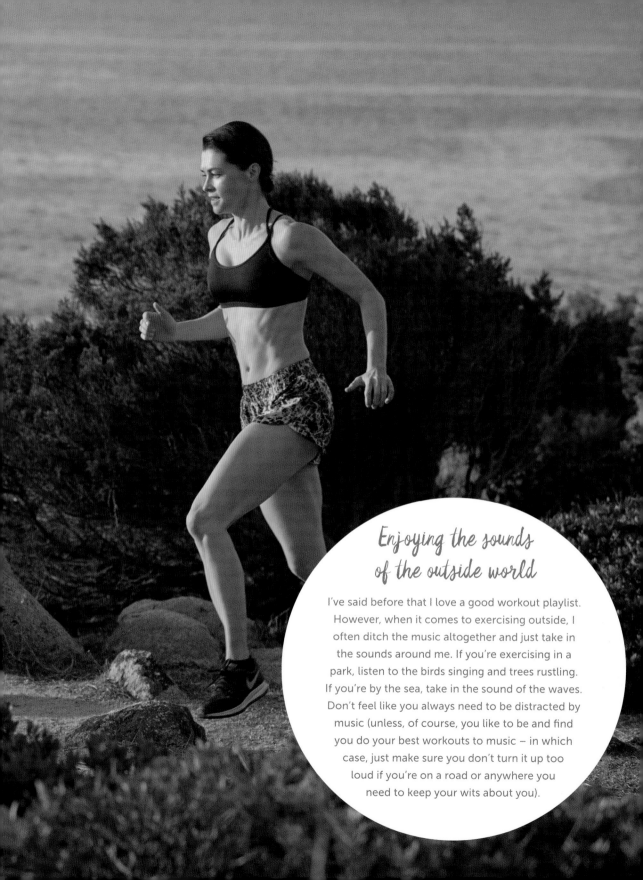

Enjoying the sounds of the outside world

I've said before that I love a good workout playlist. However, when it comes to exercising outside, I often ditch the music altogether and just take in the sounds around me. If you're exercising in a park, listen to the birds singing and trees rustling. If you're by the sea, take in the sound of the waves. Don't feel like you always need to be distracted by music (unless, of course, you like to be and find you do your best workouts to music – in which case, just make sure you don't turn it up too loud if you're on a road or anywhere you need to keep your wits about you).

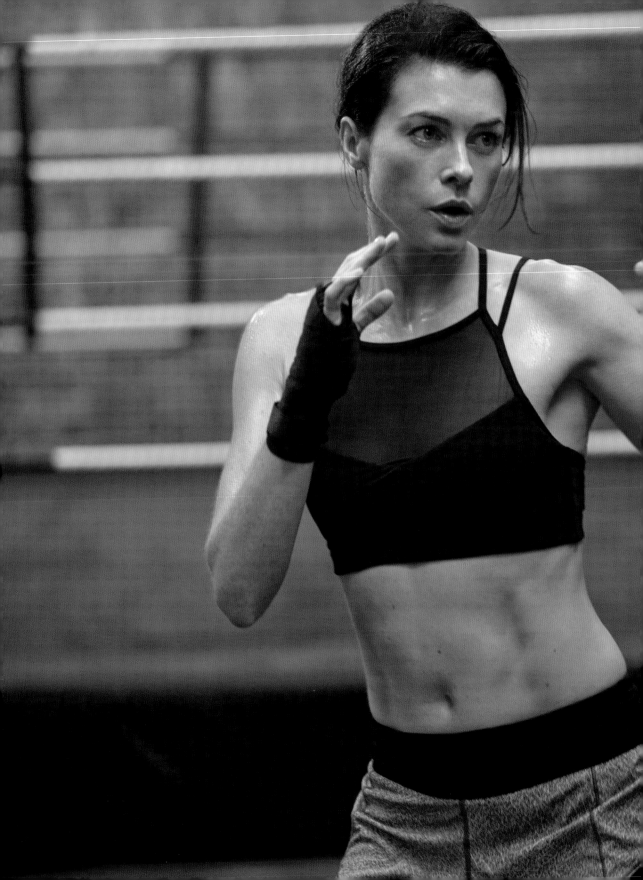

CHAPTER 4

At the Gym

I'm aware that a lot of people are wary of the gym: either they're self-conscious about exercising in front of other people, or they don't know what to do with any of the equipment so they just head to the treadmill, or they don't want the financial commitment. However, I love going to the gym. It's the best place for me to work on my strength training – a workout experience that's very hard to beat – and so I really hope that this chapter will help you to embrace it too.

If you feel self-conscious when you walk into a gym, remind yourself that everyone else is more focused on themselves and, more often than not, will be feeling a little self-conscious too. You're here for you, not for them.

If you are new to a gym, it's a good idea to keep your workouts simple to begin with. Don't overwhelm yourself with complicated exercises and don't be afraid to ask for help. A gym is an adult's playground full of amazing equipment to assist your workouts but it can be hard to know where to begin. I've given you some exercises to get you started that use minimal equipment.

Your local gym is a good place to find a personal trainer (if that's what you're after), try out a class or just change up your routine. Either way, getting to the gym once in a while is a great way to get informed and get inspired...

THE IMPORTANCE OF STRENGTH TRAINING

Strength training is a type of exercise that uses resistance (i.e. lifting, bending, pulling, pushing) to work your muscles. Examples of strength training include lifting weights, using resistance bands, using your own body weight (i.e. squats or press-ups) or using gym machines to push against (i.e. a leg curl) or pull on.

For years, there was this myth that fat burning only happened on the treadmill. However, in recent years, studies have shown that strength training is actually far more effective. In fact, a study published in the health journal *Obesity* found that, while aerobic exercises like running or cycling burn both fat and muscle, strength training burns fat alone. So rather than bulking you up (a common misconception about lifting weights), it can actually help you slim down.

This is because the body burns more calories to maintain muscle mass than it does to maintain fat. Therefore, if you build more muscle, you will raise your metabolism and burn more fat. Strength training also makes you more flexible – a study from the University of North Dakota found that it can help improve your flexibility just as well as yoga and Pilates. Strength training is also fantastic for strengthening your bones, improving joint health and it's great for your heart too. I've focused the workouts in this chapter around kettlebells and dumbbells rather than overwhelming you with lots of machines, which also means these workouts can be done anywhere.

If you're new to using weights, start light and perfect your form. Each person is unique, so there is no one size fits all answer to what weight you should use, but you do want a one that challenges you while keeping good form. These workouts combine elements of high intensity with strength training – so you'll really strengthen and tone your muscles We're hitting every muscle in the body, so get lifting.

CLAIRE, 38, PART-TIME AT AN INTERIORS DESIGN COMPANY AND MUM OF TWO

'When my youngest daughter turned two, I realised I couldn't even run up the stairs without getting out of breath. I'd had two children very close together and, while I lost my baby weight straight away, I wasn't terribly fit. I wasn't looking after myself and I didn't do any proper exercise for years.

'When I first met Holly, we started gently with squats and light weights and each week we'd build it up slowly. She also set me small challenges from week to week, like trying to fit in a swim, or go to the gym twice before I saw her again. Pretty quickly I'd caught the fitness bug. It was never about weight loss for me, and the first thing I noticed was how much stronger I felt, and more capable. I wasn't tired all the time and I literally had this spring in my step. Everything felt easier. I could be bothered to do things, whereas before everything felt like an effort. And the best thing is, I can now happily race up the stairs after my kids without getting out of breath!'

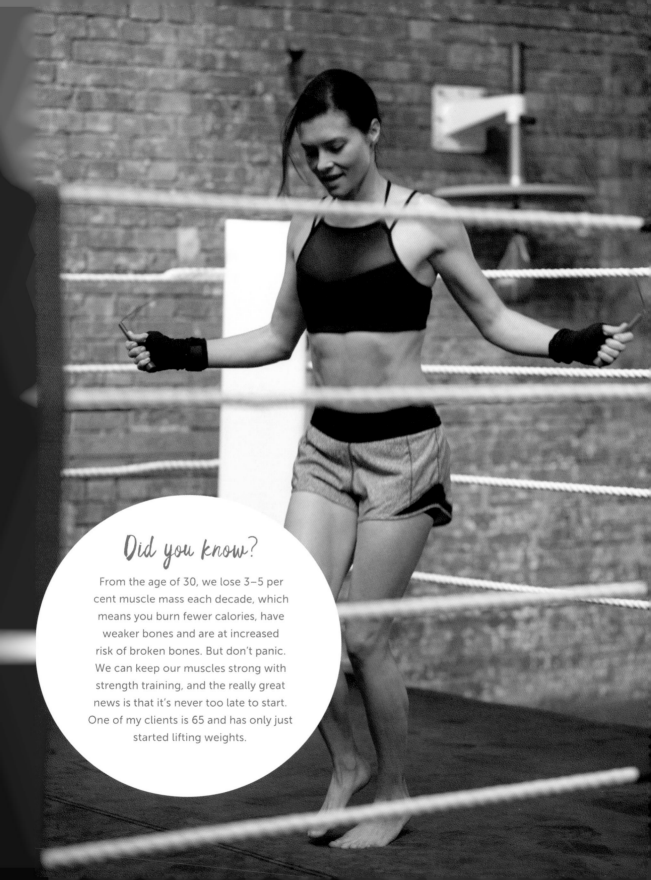

Did you know?

From the age of 30, we lose 3–5 per cent muscle mass each decade, which means you burn fewer calories, have weaker bones and are at increased risk of broken bones. But don't panic. We can keep our muscles strong with strength training, and the really great news is that it's never too late to start. One of my clients is 65 and has only just started lifting weights.

KILLER KETTLEBELL WORKOUT

This workout uses a kettlebell, but you can use a dumbbell if you prefer. A general tip for these movements – inhale when working with gravity, exhale when working against gravity (so you exhale on the effort). Perform each movement, in sequence, one after the other, with a 15 second rest between each one (if you need it). When you are done, rest for 1 minute and drink some water. Repeat the circuit 3 times, or, if you have more time or want a challenge, 4 or 5 times. As always, remember to warm up (pages 22–28) and cool down (pages 40–45).

- -

24–30 minutes (3 x 8–10 minutes)
32–40 minutes (4 x 8–10 minutes)
40–50 minutes (5 x 8–10 minutes)

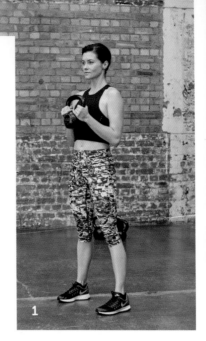

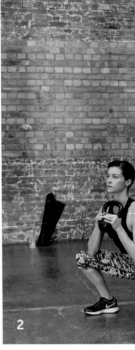

KETTLEBELL SWING

HOW TO DO IT: Stand tall with your core engaged and your feet a little wider than hip-distance apart. Hold the kettlebell handle with both hands, palms towards you, arms straight.

Maintaining a slight bend to the knee, drive the hips back, pushing your butt out behind you. Then, in a dynamic movement, drive your hips forward to swing the kettlebell into the air until your arms reach shoulder height.

With control, let the kettlebell swing back down between your legs as you bend again and keep this swinging momentum. **{15 reps}**

Don't bend too low as this isn't a squat.

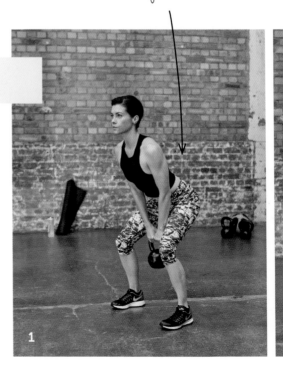

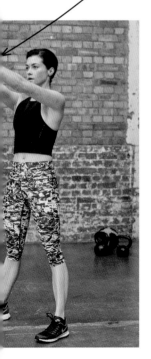

GOBLET SQUAT PRESS

HOW TO DO IT: Stand tall with your core engaged, and your feet a little wider than shoulder-width apart. Hold the kettlebell in front of your chest with cupped hands, keeping your elbows close to the body.

Keeping your back straight and chest up, start to bend your knees and move your hips slowly back and down into a squat. Keeping your weight on your heels, go as low as you can – your elbows should finish in between your knees.

Squeezing your butt cheeks and pushing back up through your heels, return to standing as you lift the kettlebell straight up over your head. With control, lower the kettlebell to chest height and repeat. **{10 reps}**

Don't try and lift the weight up – the swinging motion should be powered by your legs.

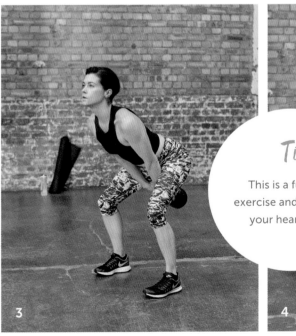

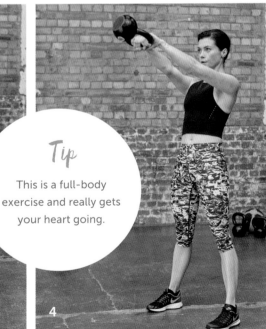

Tip

This is a full-body exercise and really gets your heart going.

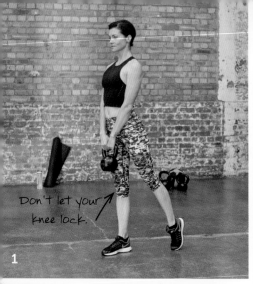

Don't let your knee lock.

1

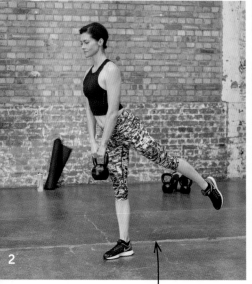

2

SINGLE LEG DEADLIFT

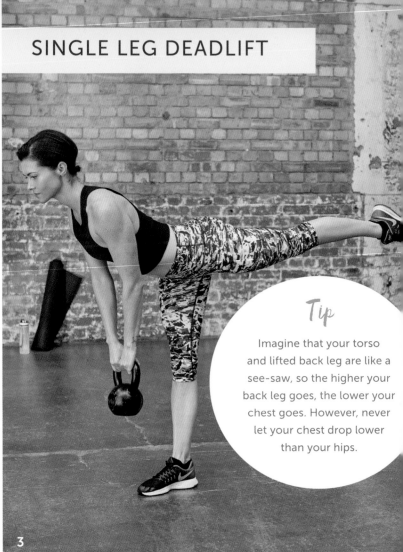

3

Tip

Imagine that your torso and lifted back leg are like a see-saw, so the higher your back leg goes, the lower your chest goes. However, never let your chest drop lower than your hips.

This could be your ending position – if you find it too difficult to bend further forward, stay here.

HOW TO DO IT: Stand tall with your core engaged and your feet a little wider than hip-distance apart. Hold the kettlebell handle with both hands, palms towards you.

Looking straight ahead, hinge at the hips and lower your torso as far forwards as you can. As you do so, slowly lift your left leg up behind you.

Lower the leg with control as you hinge the torso back up from the hips to return to the start position. Repeat with the right leg. **{10 reps each side}**

86   ACTIVE

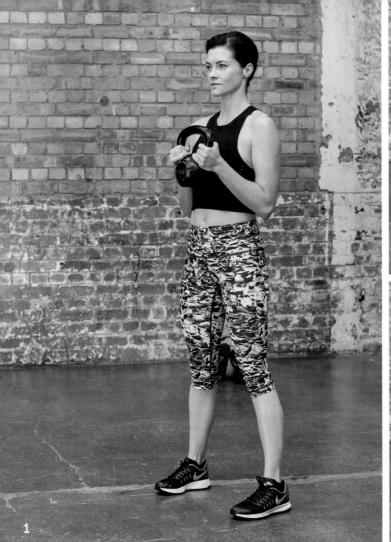

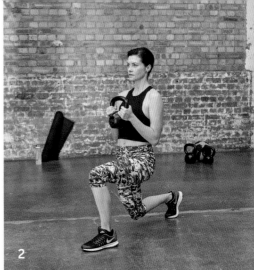

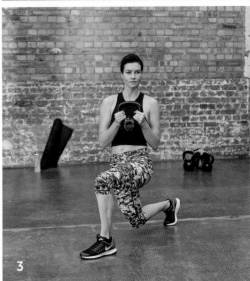

LUNGE AND ROTATE

HOW TO DO IT: Stand tall with your core engaged and your feet a little wider than hip-distance apart. Hold the kettlebell close into your chest with your elbows tucked in.

Step forward with your left leg into a lunge, getting your back knee as close to the floor as possible without it touching.

Keeping the kettlebell close to your chest, rotate your torso towards your front bent knee, then untwist and, with a big push off the front leg, return to the start position.

{10 reps each side}

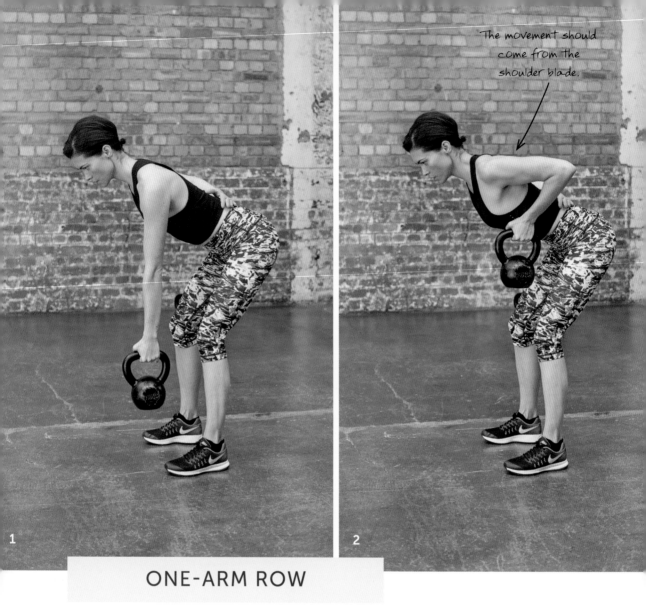

The movement should come from the shoulder blade.

1

2

ONE-ARM ROW

HOW TO DO IT: Stand tall with your core engaged and your feet a little wider than hip-distance apart. Hold a kettlebell by the handle with one hand. Lower your torso until it's almost parallel to the floor and the kettlebell hangs at arm's length from your shoulder. Rest your other arm on the small of your back. This is your start position.

Keeping your back straight and your elbow close to your side, lift the kettlebell to the side of your torso. Pause, then lower the kettlebell back to the start position with control.

{10 reps each side}

ACTIVE

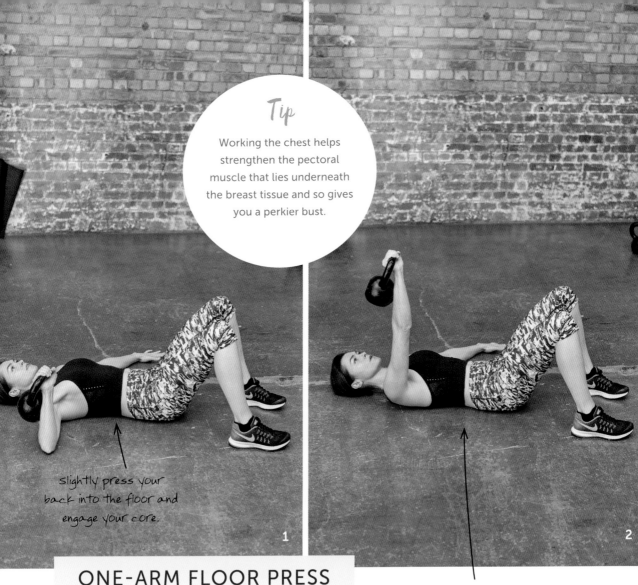

Slightly press your back into the floor and engage your core.

1

2

ONE-ARM FLOOR PRESS

As you press, you might find the opposite hip lifts due to the effort. Try to avoid this and keep your hips aligned by keeping your core engaged.

HOW TO DO IT: Lie on your back with your knees bent. Hold a kettlebell by the handle in one hand with your elbow in line with your shoulder at 90 degrees.

Press the weight straight up towards the ceiling. Pause at the top.

Lower the kettlebell back to the start position with control and repeat. **{10 reps each side}**

DUMBBELL DYNAMO

Perform each movement, in sequence, one after the other. Ideally, don't rest until the end but, if you need to, take a little break between each exercise. When you are done, rest for 1 minute, drink some water, then repeat the circuit 3 times. If you have more time or want a challenge, repeat 4 or 5 times.

- - - - - - - - - - - - - - - - - - -

18 minutes (3 x 6 minutes)
24 minutes (4 x 6 minutes)
30 minutes (5 x 6 minutes)

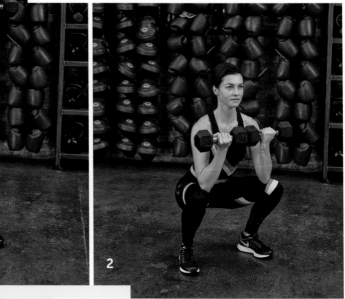

FRONT SQUAT

HOW TO DO IT: Stand tall with your core engaged and feet shoulder-width apart. Hold a dumbbell in each hand, palms facing towards you, hugging them close to your chest.

Keeping your back straight and your chest high, squat down until the crease of the hip drops below the level of the knee.

Pause at the bottom, then push your weight into the floor and drive off your heels to return to the start position. **{10 reps}**

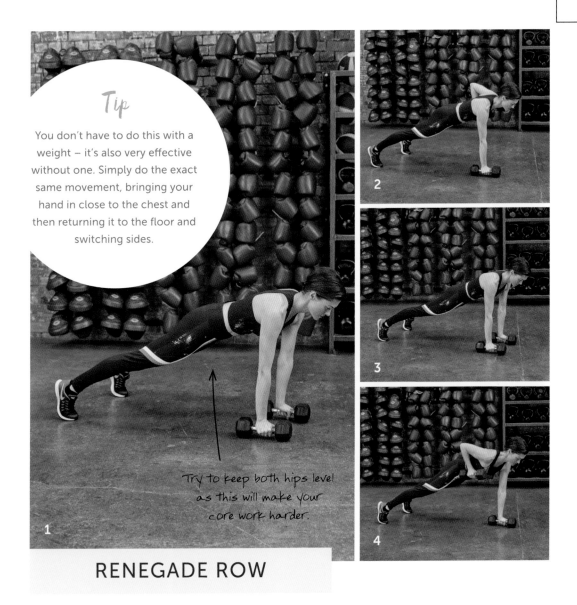

Tip

You don't have to do this with a weight – it's also very effective without one. Simply do the exact same movement, bringing your hand in close to the chest and then returning it to the floor and switching sides.

Try to keep both hips level as this will make your core work harder.

1

2

3

4

RENEGADE ROW

HOW TO DO IT: Grab a pair of dumbbells and get into a high plank position with your hands on the weights and feet hip-width apart.

Pulling from your shoulder blades, bend one elbow in a rowing action to bring the dumbbell close to your chest.

Return the dumbbell to the floor with control and keep alternating sides. **{20 reps total}**

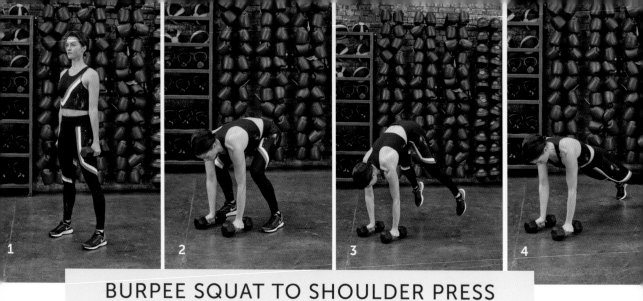

BURPEE SQUAT TO SHOULDER PRESS

HOW TO DO IT: Holding a dumbbell in each hand, stand tall, core engaged, with your arms by your sides and feet about hip-width apart.

Squat down and rest the dumbbells on the floor, then jump both feet back into a high plank position. Immediately jump them forwards again, and then return to standing.

As you stand, bring the dumbbells up to your shoulders.

Lift the dumbbells above your head until your arms are straight, then lower the weights back down to the start position. Repeat. **{10 reps}**

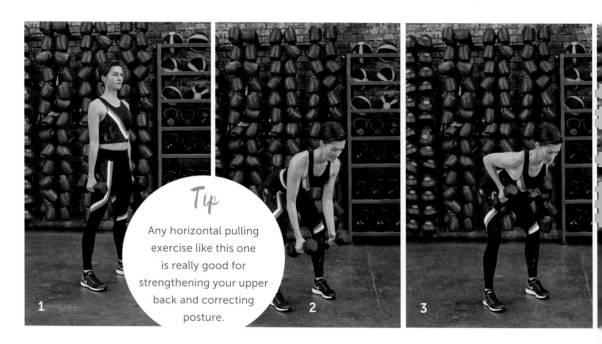

Tip

Any horizontal pulling exercise like this one is really good for strengthening your upper back and correcting posture.

ACTIVE

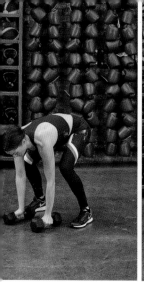

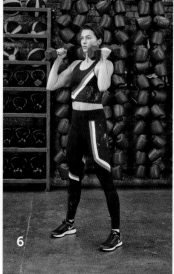

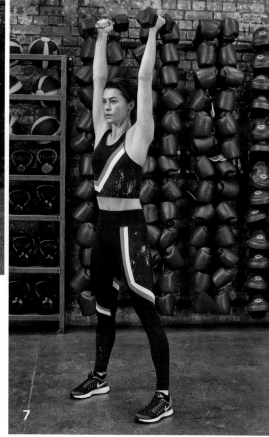

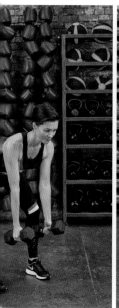

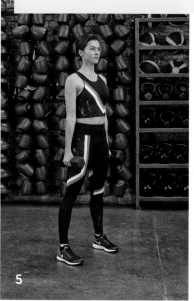

BENT OVER ROW TO DEADLIFT

HOW TO DO IT: With a dumbbell in each hand, stand tall, core engaged, with your feet shoulder-width apart and knees slightly bent.

Keeping your navel drawn in so your core is engaged and your back straight, sit your hips back to lower your torso towards the floor, letting your arms hang down. Squeeze your shoulder blades together and pull the weights up to your ribs.

Slowly lower the dumbbells with control and, slightly pushing your hips forwards and squeezing your butt cheeks, come up to standing with a straight back. Finish with knees slightly bent and repeat. **{10 reps}**

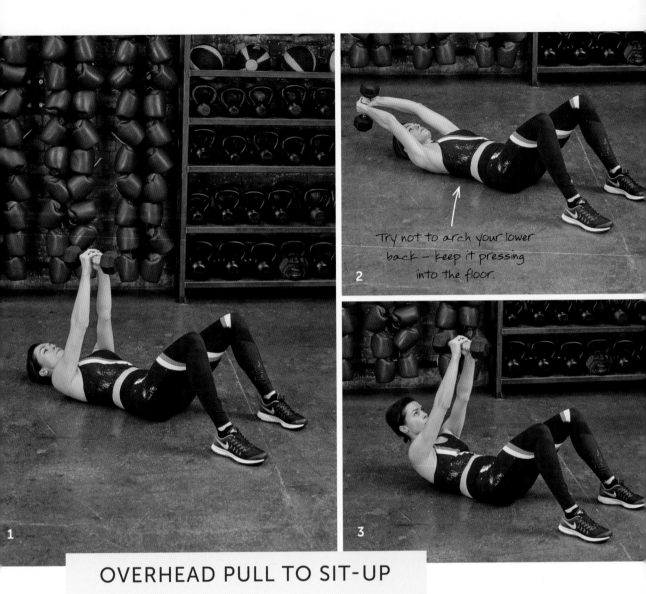

Try not to arch your lower back – keep it pressing into the floor.

OVERHEAD PULL TO SIT-UP

HOW TO DO IT: Lie on your back with your knees bent and feet hip-width apart. Slightly press your lower back into the floor and engage your core. Hold a dumbbell in both hands with your arms straight, above your chest. Keeping your arms straight, lower them behind your head until they nearly touch the floor. Keeping your core engaged, lift the dumbbell until it's directly above your chest and, lifting only your shoulder blades off the floor, raise your upper body in a 'sit-up'.

Slowly lower your upper body back to the floor and return your arms to behind your head.
{10 reps}

ACTIVE

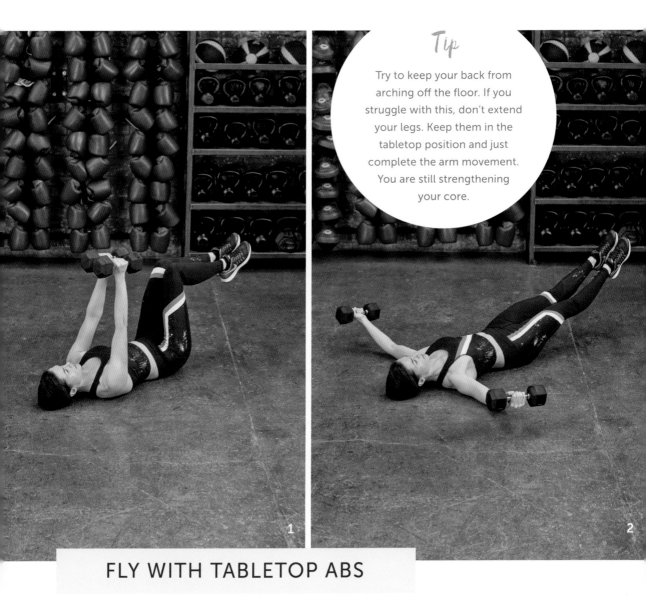

Tip

Try to keep your back from arching off the floor. If you struggle with this, don't extend your legs. Keep them in the tabletop position and just complete the arm movement. You are still strengthening your core.

1

2

FLY WITH TABLETOP ABS

HOW TO DO IT: Lie on your back, bend your legs and lift your knees up into a tabletop position, so your shins are parallel to the ceiling. Holding a dumbbell in each hand, raise your arms towards the ceiling, with your palms facing each other and your elbows slightly bent.

Keeping your torso stable, open your arms out to the sides until your elbows are about 2cm from the floor. At the same time, extend your legs out.

Keeping your core engaged, return to the start position. **{10 reps}**

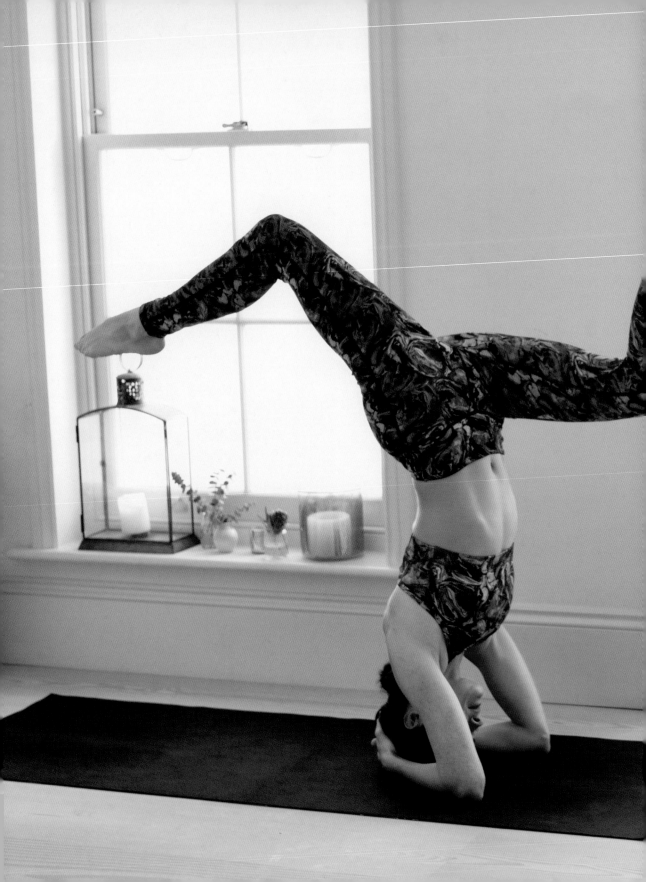

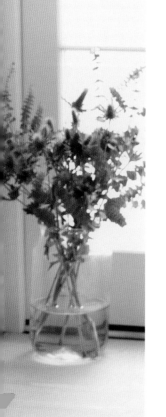

CHAPTER 5

In the Studio

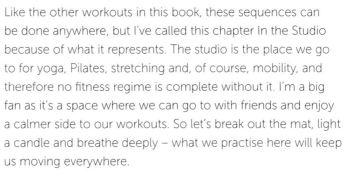

Like the other workouts in this book, these sequences can be done anywhere, but I've called this chapter In the Studio because of what it represents. The studio is the place we go to for yoga, Pilates, stretching and, of course, mobility, and therefore no fitness regime is complete without it. I'm a big fan as it's a space where we can go to with friends and enjoy a calmer side to our workouts. So let's break out the mat, light a candle and breathe deeply – what we practise here will keep us moving everywhere.

Mobility is the bedrock of good health, and keeping yourself mobile should be the foundation of your fitness. It helps you stand taller with better posture and will ensure you're as fit, healthy and agile as possible, long into old age. I always tell clients that if they stay mobile they won't have trouble getting out of chairs or bending down to tie up their shoelaces when they get older because their bodies will be a lot less stiff.

The common mistake people often make with their fitness, especially in their twenties and thirties when the body has a lot of natural flexibility anyway, is to overlook mobility and focus purely on cardio or strength training. Stretching should be a key component of any workout and, especially as you get older, good mobility makes every other exercise, like running, squats and lifting weights, that much easier.

WHAT IS MOBILITY?

In basic terms, it's our ability to move our body freely without pain or stiffness. Mobility training – in other words, exercises like yoga and Pilates – can improve this ability and our range of movements. It helps with our posture, our ability to touch our toes and enables us to move our body in the ways it is designed to move. Plus it can ward off lower-back pain or niggling joint problems like creaky knees or stiff shoulders.

Furthermore, aside from the physical benefits, mobility exercises like yoga and Pilates are invaluable when it comes to managing stress. For me, yoga is like exercise for my mind. It's not about getting my heart rate up or burning calories, but rather quietening that chatter we all get in our heads when we lead busy lives and controlling our breathing, which always leaves us happier and calmer.

I grew up working on my mobility thanks to my yoga-loving mum and big sister, Sadie. But it's never too late to start improving your mobility. I know men and women in their sixties who suddenly take up Pilates, having never done anything like it before. So aim to do at least one move a day, or a few moves every week and build from there.

A WORD ON BREATHING

The average person breathes in and out more than 23,000 times a day and, for many of us, it's just a thoughtless action. However, our breathing can have a huge impact on how we feel. Many of my clients do what I call 'stress breathing', where they're almost too busy to breathe properly and take quick or shallow breaths. This can cause a raised heart rate, raised cortisol levels (the stress hormone) and create tension in the body. Becoming a better breather can therefore pay off hugely in terms of health and wellness. And the best thing is, it's free and easy and you can do it anywhere.

So how can you breathe better? For a start, become more aware of your own breathing. If you're stressed or in a rush, or totally wrapped up in your work (especially if you have a sedentary, office-based job) you'll probably notice how shallow your breathing can get at times. So every once in a while, throughout the day, place your hand on your stomach and breathe in deeply through your nose – not your mouth – so your stomach and chest puff out with air. Hold for a few moments, then release through your nose or mouth until your stomach and chest flatten.

Do it once or twice, or until you feel a little calmer and refreshed. You'll notice that the effect is instantaneous. I often do this if I'm stuck in a traffic jam or just feeling a little overwhelmed. Or sometimes I do it simply to 'reset' and focus my mind.

Tip

If you need to take a pause at any point during these workouts, come into child's pose for a few moments (page 19).

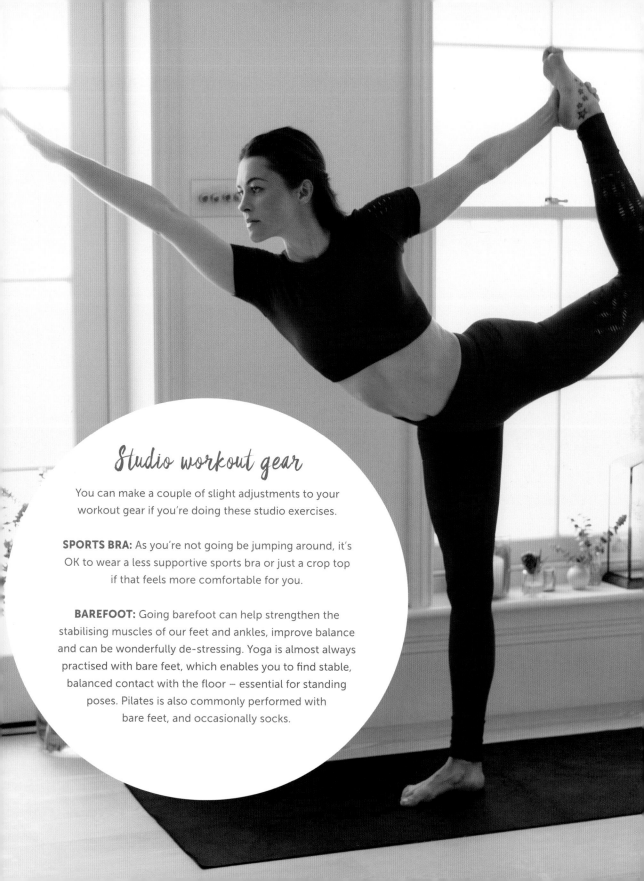

Studio workout gear

You can make a couple of slight adjustments to your workout gear if you're doing these studio exercises.

SPORTS BRA: As you're not going be jumping around, it's OK to wear a less supportive sports bra or just a crop top if that feels more comfortable for you.

BAREFOOT: Going barefoot can help strengthen the stabilising muscles of our feet and ankles, improve balance and can be wonderfully de-stressing. Yoga is almost always practised with bare feet, which enables you to find stable, balanced contact with the floor – essential for standing poses. Pilates is also commonly performed with bare feet, and occasionally socks.

STRENGTHEN & LENGTHEN

YOGA-STYLE WORKOUT

We're working on mobility here. Pay attention to your alignment and your breathing. Getting the breathing right will really benefit you. Try not to overthink it, but aim to exhale on the effort. This sequence is very grounding and a great way to feel balanced and centred. Take your time. Do each exercise one after the other. Rest in child's pose and repeat.

- -

16–20 MINUTES (2 X 6–8 MINUTES)

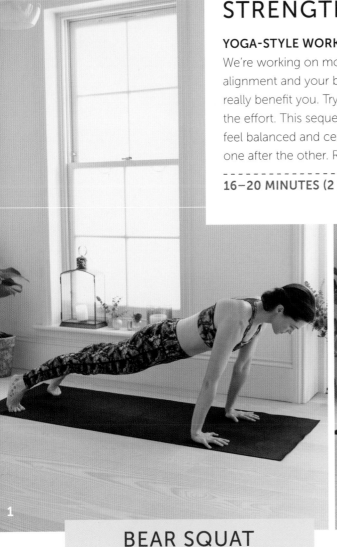

1

BEAR SQUAT

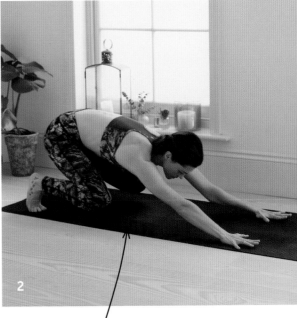

2

Inhale as you shift your weight backwards, exhale as you drive forwards.

HOW TO DO IT: Start in a high plank position with shoulders directly over your wrists, keeping a straight line from your head to your heels. Bend your knees and push your butt back towards your heels, keeping your knees off the floor.

Push into the feet, driving forwards and returning to plank. **{5 reps}**

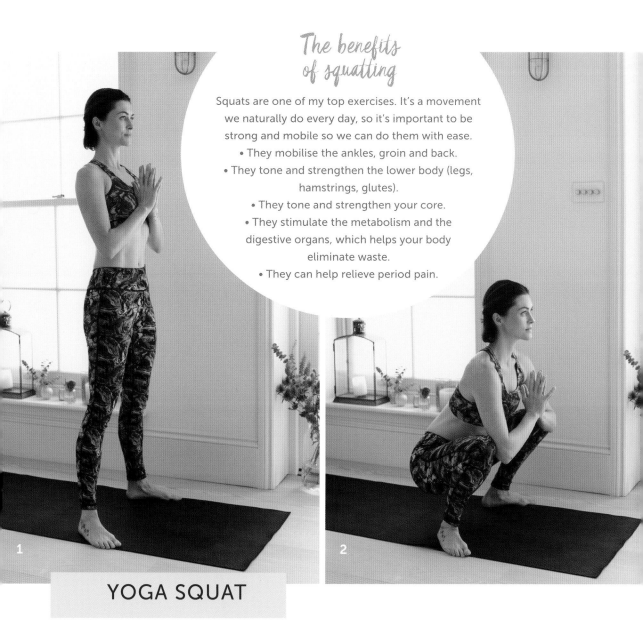

The benefits of squatting

Squats are one of my top exercises. It's a movement we naturally do every day, so it's important to be strong and mobile so we can do them with ease.

• They mobilise the ankles, groin and back.
• They tone and strengthen the lower body (legs, hamstrings, glutes).
• They tone and strengthen your core.
• They stimulate the metabolism and the digestive organs, which helps your body eliminate waste.
• They can help relieve period pain.

YOGA SQUAT

HOW TO DO IT: Stand tall, core engaged, with your feet just wider than hip-width apart and your toes turned out slightly. Bring your palms together at your heart centre.

Bend your knees to lower your butt as far as you can. You can use your elbows to push your knees out. Relax in this position for 2–3 breaths.

Keeping your chest lifted and your back straight, engage your core and push down through your heels to stand back up. **{10 reps}**

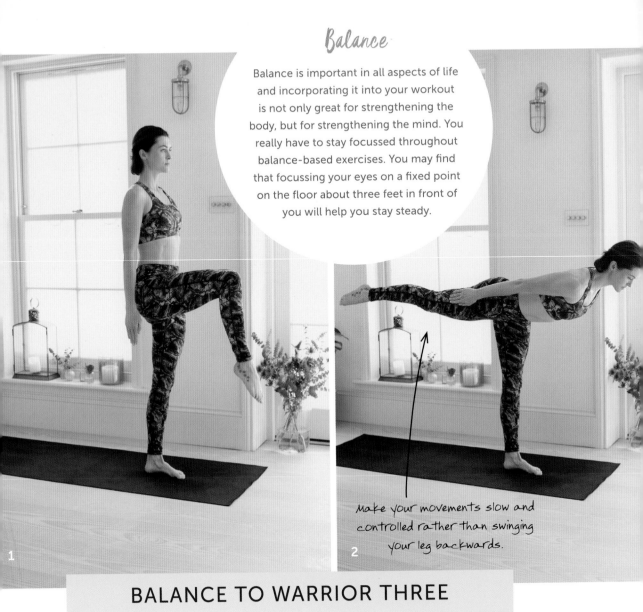

Balance

Balance is important in all aspects of life and incorporating it into your workout is not only great for strengthening the body, but for strengthening the mind. You really have to stay focussed throughout balance-based exercises. You may find that focussing your eyes on a fixed point on the floor about three feet in front of you will help you stay steady.

Make your movements slow and controlled rather than swinging your leg backwards.

1

2

BALANCE TO WARRIOR THREE

HOW TO DO IT: Stand with your arms by your sides and feet shoulder-width apart. Lift your right leg, bending at the knee to a 90-degree angle and keeping your left foot firmly rooted.

Extend the right leg straight back behind you, hinging at the hips and, keeping your arms straight at your side, let your torso come forward to form a straight line with your raised leg. WIthout letting your right foot touch the floor, bring it back to the standing balance with your knee at 90 degrees. **{10 reps each side.}**

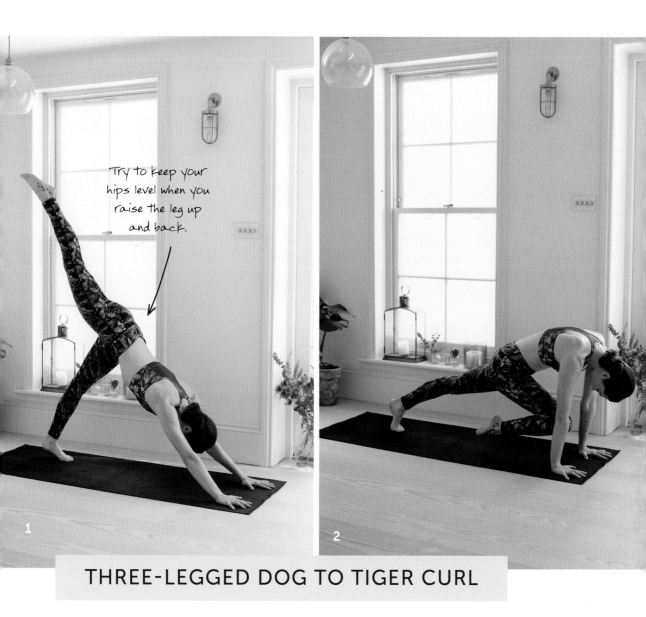

Try to keep your hips level when you raise the leg up and back.

THREE-LEGGED DOG TO TIGER CURL

HOW TO DO IT: Start in downward dog (page 25) and lift your right leg straight up into the air (three-legged dog).

As you shift your shoulders forwards over your wrists and come into a plank position, sweep your right leg forwards, bending it at the knee and tucking it into your chest. Draw in your core (hollowing your stomach) as you hold this pose.

Push back into three-legged dog and repeat without your right foot coming back to the floor.
{5 reps each side}

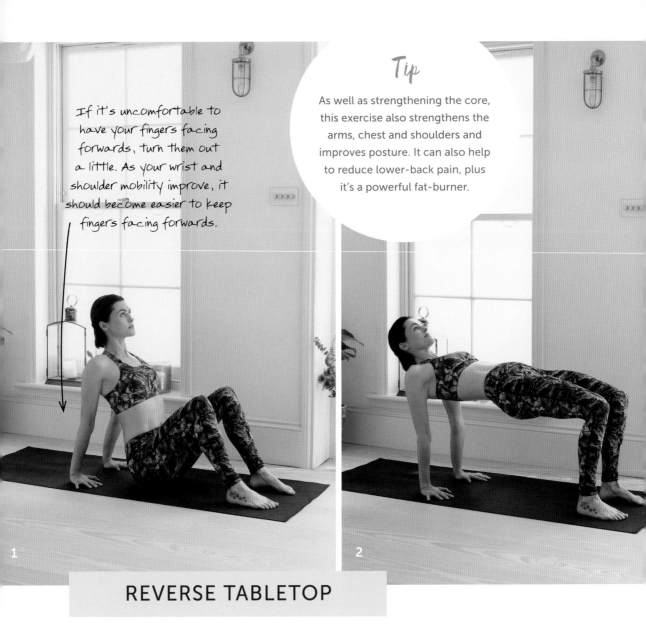

If it's uncomfortable to have your fingers facing forwards, turn them out a little. As your wrist and shoulder mobility improve, it should become easier to keep fingers facing forwards.

Tip

As well as strengthening the core, this exercise also strengthens the arms, chest and shoulders and improves posture. It can also help to reduce lower-back pain, plus it's a powerful fat-burner.

1

2

REVERSE TABLETOP

HOW TO DO IT: Sit with your knees bent and your hands on the floor directly under your shoulders, fingers facing forwards.

Driving your heels and palms into the ground, lift your hips towards the ceiling until your body forms a table, with your stomach parallel to the ceiling. Engage your core and squeeze your glutes to hold the position for 3 breaths.

With control, lower your butt down to touch the floor. **{5 reps}**

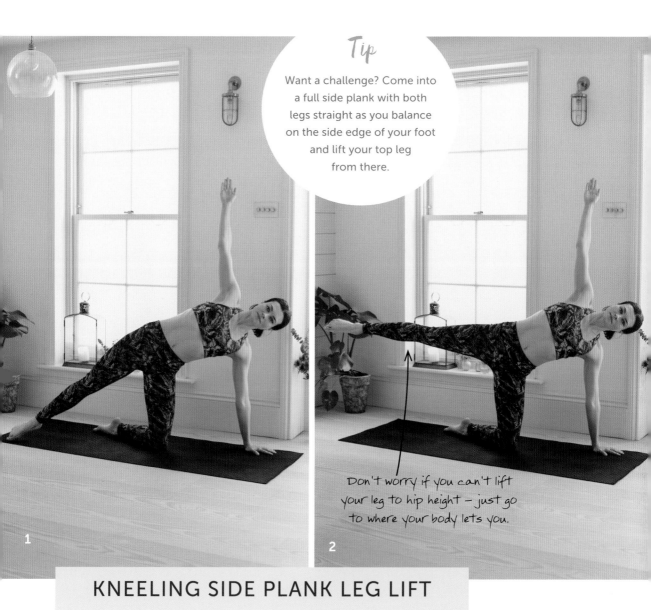

Tip

Want a challenge? Come into a full side plank with both legs straight as you balance on the side edge of your foot and lift your top leg from there.

Don't worry if you can't lift your leg to hip height — just go to where your body lets you.

1

2

KNEELING SIDE PLANK LEG LIFT

HOW TO DO IT: Come into a kneeling side plank position, with your left hand under your shoulder and your left knee under your hip. Raise your right arm towards the ceiling.

Keeping your core engaged and your right leg straight, slowly lift it to hip height, then lower it back down with control. **{10 reps each side}**

INNER CORE FOCUS

PILATES-STYLE WORKOUT

This is a full body workout with extra focus on your core. Take your time and make slow, controlled movements. Keep coming back to your core, making sure it's engaged.

16–20 MINUTES (2 X 6–8 MINUTES)

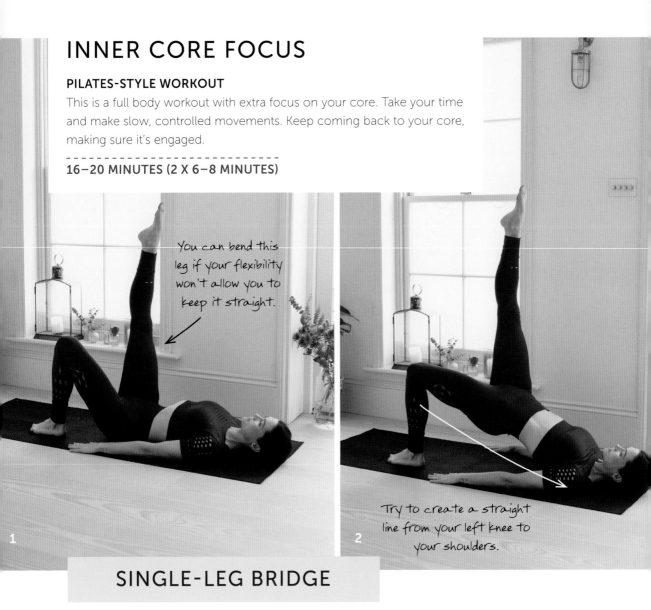

You can bend this leg if your flexibility won't allow you to keep it straight.

Try to create a straight line from your left knee to your shoulders.

1

2

SINGLE-LEG BRIDGE

HOW TO DO IT: Lie on your back with your hands by your sides, both knees bent and your feet flat on the floor. Make sure your feet are under your knees. Extend the right leg straight up.

Engaging your core and squeezing your butt muscles, press down with the left foot to drive your hips up to a bridge position.

Lower the hips back to the floor. Keep your right leg raised as you repeat the movement.

{10 reps each side}

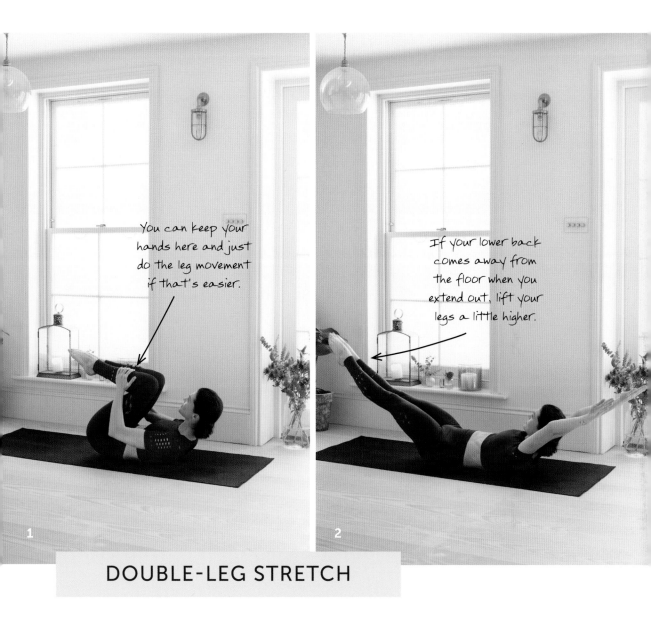

You can keep your hands here and just do the leg movement if that's easier.

If your lower back comes away from the floor when you extend out, lift your legs a little higher.

1

2

DOUBLE-LEG STRETCH

HOW TO DO IT: Lie on your back, with knees bent at a 90-degree angle and your hands resting on your shins. Your lower back should be pressed against the floor and your head, neck and shoulders should be slightly raised off the mat.

Keeping your core engaged (navel drawn in towards your spine), simultaneously straighten your legs and stretch your arms straight behind your head.

Reverse the motion, returning to the start position. **{10 reps}**

PLANK ROTATION

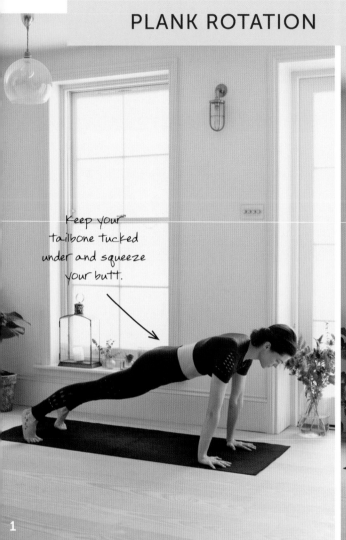

Keep your tailbone tucked under and squeeze your butt.

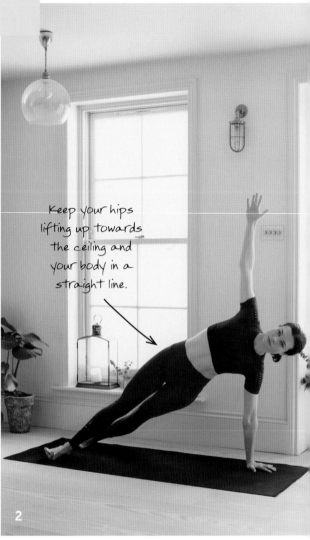

Keep your hips lifting up towards the ceiling and your body in a straight line.

HOW TO DO IT: Start in a plank position with hands and elbows under your shoulders, your neck in line with your spine and your feet a little wider than hip-width apart.

In one, controlled move, extend the right arm straight above your head as you rotate the torso, coming onto the sides of your feet. Hold for 2–3 breaths.

Return to a plank position and repeat on the other side. **{10 reps in total}**

DONKEY KICK

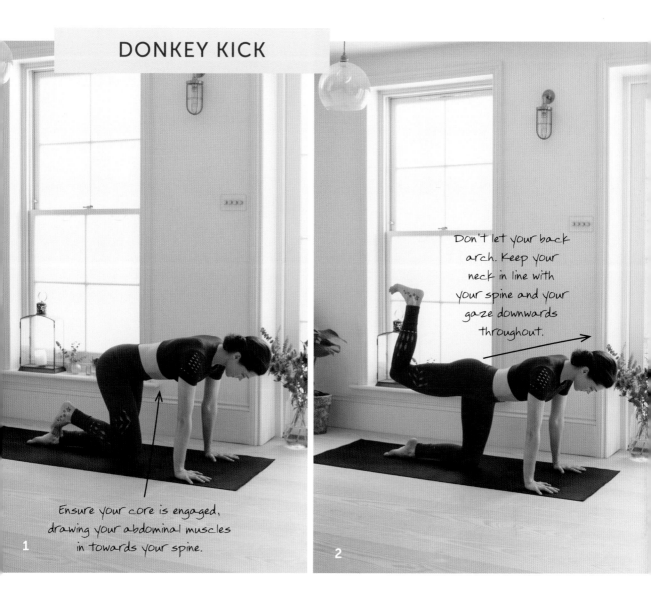

Ensure your core is engaged, drawing your abdominal muscles in towards your spine.

1

Don't let your back arch. Keep your neck in line with your spine and your gaze downwards throughout.

2

HOW TO DO IT: Begin on all fours, knees hip-width apart, hands directly under your shoulders and your head and spine in a straight line.

Flex your right foot and, using your glutes, drive the leg back as high as it can go, keeping your knee bent, while your pelvis and hips stay parallel to the floor.

Pause for one breath and then repeat. **{10 reps each side}**

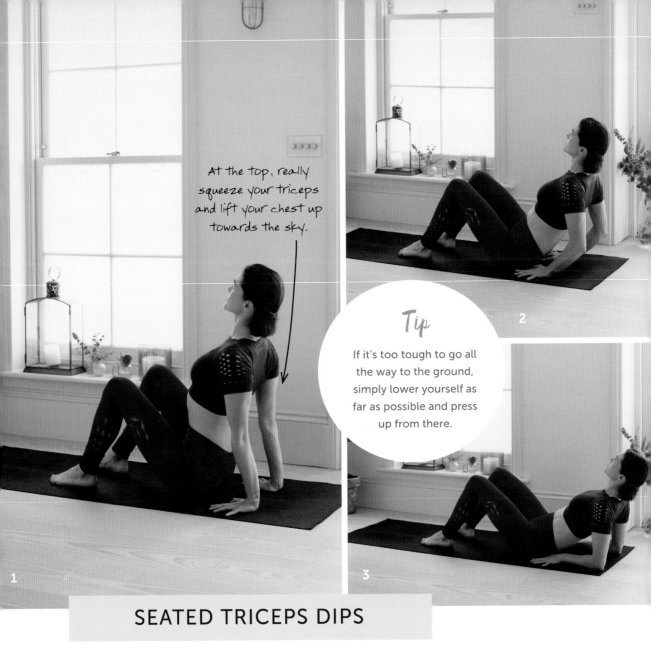

At the top, really squeeze your triceps and lift your chest up towards the sky.

Tip

If it's too tough to go all the way to the ground, simply lower yourself as far as possible and press up from there.

1

2

3

SEATED TRICEPS DIPS

HOW TO DO IT: Sit with your knees bent and your hands behind you with your fingers facing forwards. Bending the elbows, slowly lower yourself back until your forearms rest on the floor. Press into the hands to push yourself back up into the starting position. **{10 reps}**

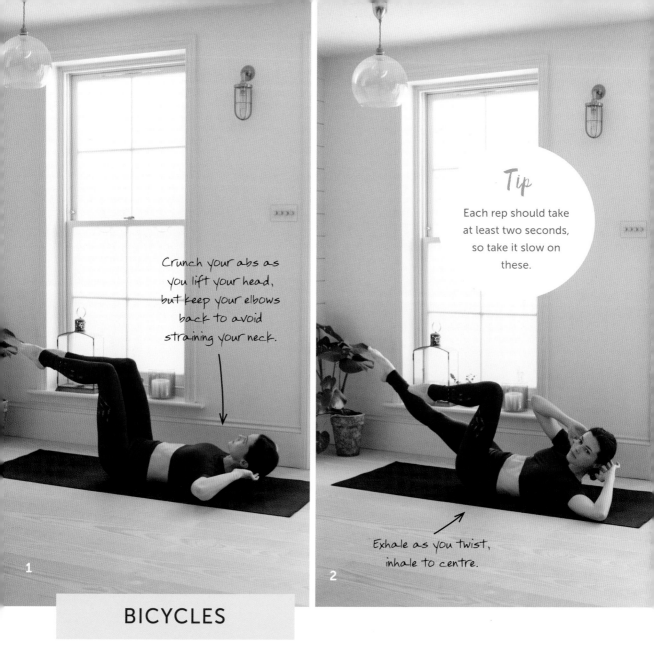

Crunch your abs as you lift your head, but keep your elbows back to avoid straining your neck.

Tip
Each rep should take at least two seconds, so take it slow on these.

Exhale as you twist, inhale to centre.

1

2

BICYCLES

HOW TO DO IT: Lie on your back with your hands behind your head, supporting your neck with your fingers. Engage your core and push the small of your back against the floor and bring your knees into a tabletop position (see **1**).

Pull your left knee in towards your chest while also lifting your shoulder blades off the floor, rotating the torso and bringing the right elbow towards the left knee. Lift your head a little to touch the elbow to the knee. Return to tabletop and then switch sides, extending the left leg as you bend the right knee and lift the left elbow.

Alternate each side in a pedalling motion, using slow, controlled movements. **{10 reps total}**

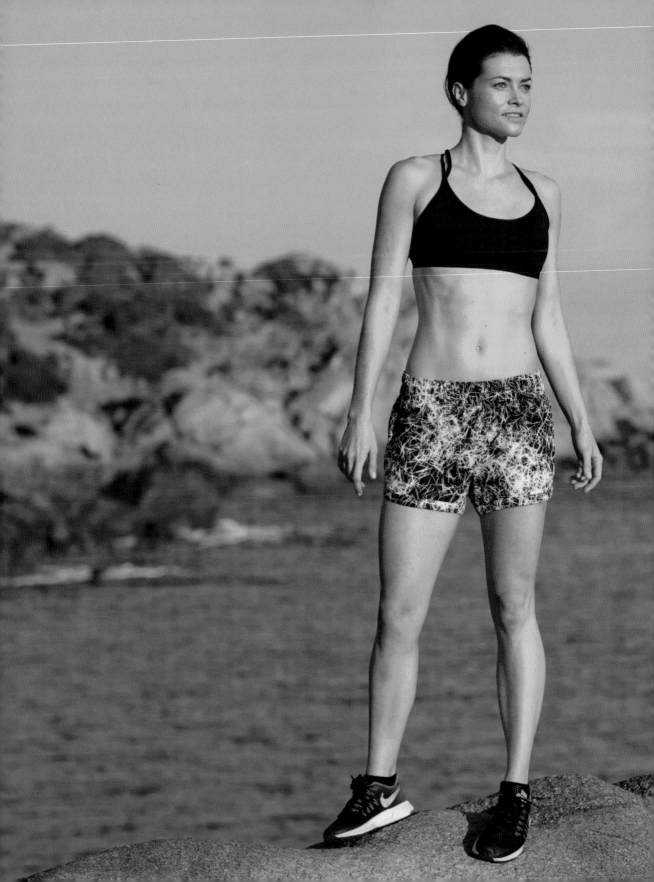

CHAPTER 6

On Holiday

Everyone overindulges on holiday. Working out just a little can really counteract that – and feeling more in tune with your body can help you avoid overdoing it in the first place. There's no need to stop exercising when you go on holiday – keep up with your routine while you're away and you'll find it easier to carry on with it when you get back. This is a lifestyle, after all. In fact, I often find I exercise more when I'm away because I have more time, am less stressed and have access to great locations, like the beach, new bike trails or fantastic coastal walks. Walking, running or hiking are great ways to explore a new place, while also accomplishing a satisfying workout.

So what can you look out for while you're away?

STAND-UP PADDLE BOARDING (known as SUP Boarding)

This was first practised by Hawaiians and is now the world's fastest-growing watersport, popular everywhere from the US to the UK. As the name suggests, it involves standing up on a surfboard and paddling and, because you have to really use your core to keep you upright, it provides the perfect core workout, plus it's a lot of fun.

SUP BOARD YOGA

This is similar to the above, but it involves doing yoga moves on the board, which becomes like a floating yoga mat! And because it's floating, this provides another fantastic workout for your core because you have to work harder to stay stable and upright. It's probably not one for beginners though and is best suited to people with experience of either yoga or SUP Boarding.

HIKING

The trend for hiking and trekking on holiday is huge, especially in places like Los Angeles. All you need is a pair of sensible shoes (either trainers or hiking boots), a bottle of water, a packed lunch and a good map and you're set up for an adventure.

SWIMMING

Swimming is a simple but really underrated holiday workout. It provides an all-over body workout and yet it's low impact so really kind on the joints, and it boosts your mood and helps you sleep.

ROCK CLIMBING

It's best to do this under the supervision and care of a professional rock-climbing instructor. It provides a great cardio and strength training workout for both the upper and lower body, and it can boost confidence and reduce stress.

HOLIDAY WORKOUT TIPS

Holidays are about exploring somewhere new. As unfamiliar environments can throw up a few surprises, here are a few tips that hopefully mean you're always prepared.

- Wear the right clothing: wicking fitness clothing is lightweight and breathable and keeps you cool.
- If you're in a very hot country, find cool places to exercise in, like shady woods or breezy shorelines. Don't, of course, exercise without sun protection, and avoid the harsh midday sun. Exercise early in the morning or late afternoon/ evening when the sun is less intense.
- Keep it short (if you want to). If you're keen to relax and make the most of your holiday, squeeze in a little fitness 'snack' and just do ten minutes. That ten minutes will still make a difference to your fitness levels – and you may find (as I often do) that you want to carry on for a little longer. And if you don't, you can still feel proud.
- Use your surroundings: if you have a pool at your hotel or villa, swim a few lengths. If there's a steep cliff face up from the beach, power walk up it. Use nature as your gym.

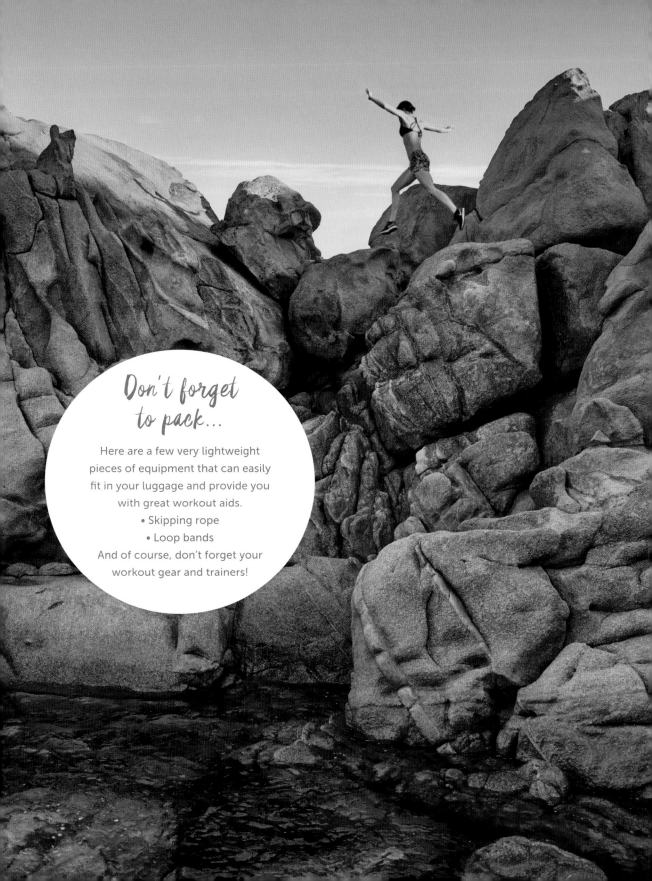

Don't forget to pack...

Here are a few very lightweight pieces of equipment that can easily fit in your luggage and provide you with great workout aids.

- Skipping rope
- Loop bands

And of course, don't forget your workout gear and trainers!

SUNSHINE WORKOUT

If you're hotel-bound (especially if you're travelling for work), here are some holiday-themed exercises to try the next time you go away. However, as well as your hotel room or hotel gym, you can also do them on the beach, in a city park or anywhere else you like. Remember – you're on holiday, so let's keep this short and speedy. Whizz through this workout twice, then enjoy the sunshine.

----

16 MINUTES (2 X 8 MINUTES)

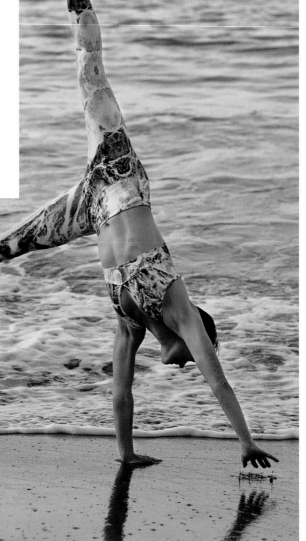

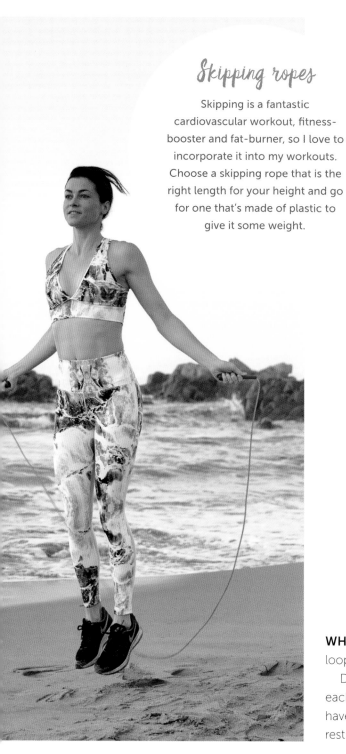

Skipping ropes

Skipping is a fantastic cardiovascular workout, fitness-booster and fat-burner, so I love to incorporate it into my workouts. Choose a skipping rope that is the right length for your height and go for one that's made of plastic to give it some weight.

Workout summary

Just in case you can't take your book with you on holiday, here's a quick breakdown of this workout – take a snapshot on your phone and you're good to go.

Skip 30 seconds
Rest 15 seconds
Sundial Lunge (left) 30 seconds
Sundial Lunge (right) 30 seconds
Skip 30 seconds
Rest 15 seconds
Crab toe touch 30 seconds
Skip 30 seconds
Rest 15 seconds
Prone swimming 30 seconds
Skip 30 seconds
Rest 15 seconds
Plank push ups 30 seconds
Skip 30 seconds
Rest 15 seconds
Tummy tightener 30 seconds
Repeat from top.

If you want more of a challenge, miss out the rests.

You'll find summaries of every workout in the book on pages 168–170.

WHAT DO I NEED?: A skipping rope and a loop band.

Do 30 seconds of skipping in between each exercise (or jog on the spot if you don't have a skipping rope) and take a 15-second rest each time before you move on.

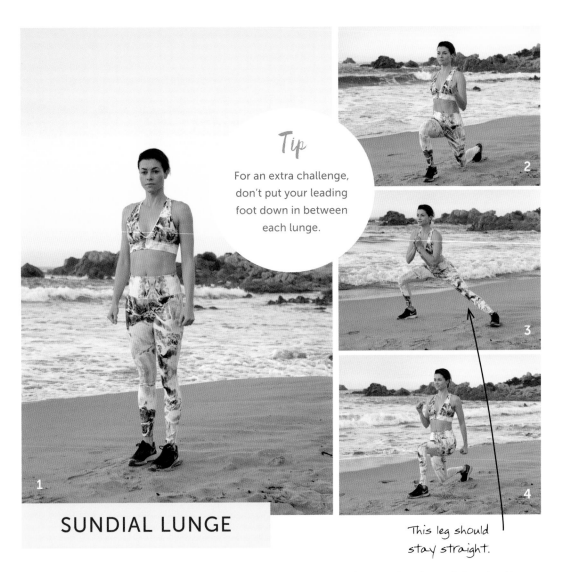

Tip

For an extra challenge, don't put your leading foot down in between each lunge.

This leg should stay straight.

SUNDIAL LUNGE

HOW TO DO IT: This exercise involves performing a series of lunges in a 'round-the-clock' movement. Stand tall with your core engaged. Lunge forwards with your right foot and lower until your right knee forms a 90-degree angle. Make sure your front knee is directly above your ankle. Driving off your front heel, return to standing.

Take a big step or lunge out to your right with your right leg, your left leg staying straight. Again, driving off the right heel, return to standing.

Finally, lunge backwards with your right leg so that your left and right knees each form a 90-degree angle. Again, drive off the heel to return to standing.

Repeat for 30 seconds, then do the same with the other leg. **{30 seconds each leg, then skip for 30 seconds}**

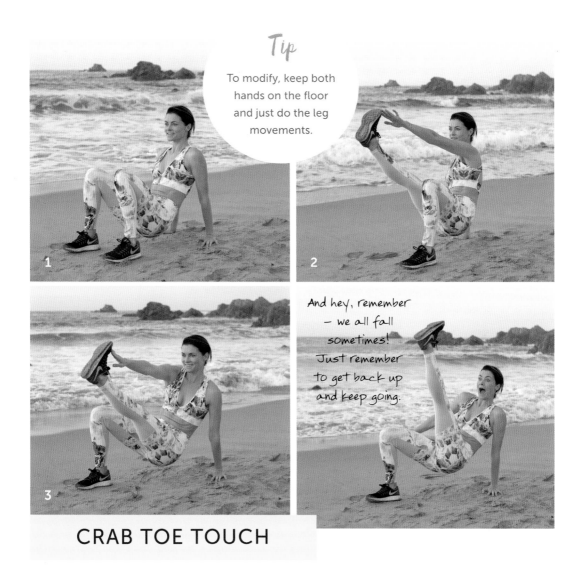

Tip

To modify, keep both hands on the floor and just do the leg movements.

And hey, remember — we all fall sometimes! Just remember to get back up and keep going.

CRAB TOE TOUCH

HOW TO DO IT: Sit with your knees bent, feet apart and your hands flat on the ground behind you. Lift your butt off the floor.

Kick your right leg straight up and try to touch your toes with your left hand.

Return your right foot to the ground, kick your left leg straight up and try to touch your toes with your right hand.

Keep alternating sides for 30 seconds. **{30 seconds total, then skip for 30 seconds}**

PRONE SWIMMING

HOW TO DO IT: Lie face-down with your core engaged, legs straight and arms reaching overhead.

Lift one leg and the opposite arm upwards, then lower and switch over to the other side quickly, without losing balance in the centre of your torso.

Keep going for 30 seconds. **{30 seconds total, then skip for 30 seconds}**

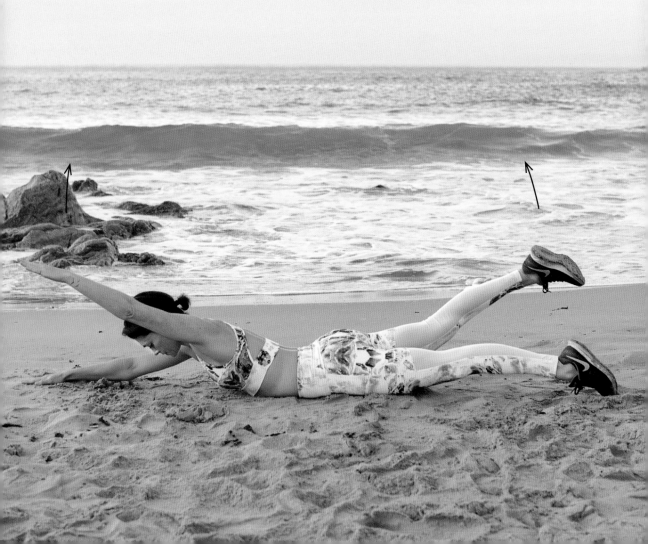

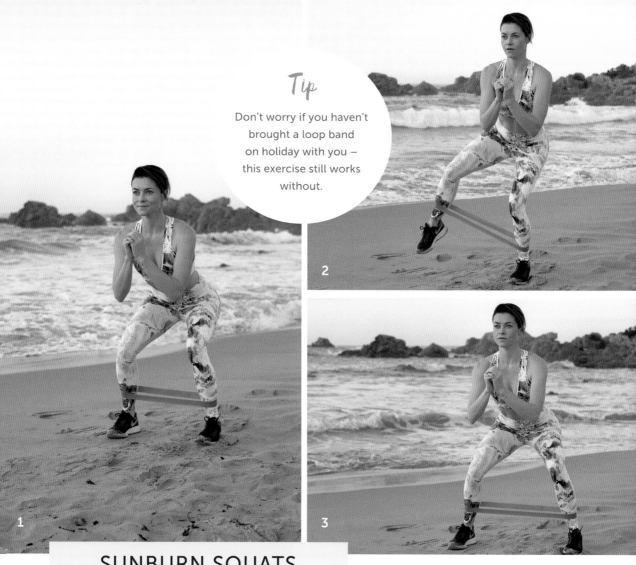

Tip

Don't worry if you haven't brought a loop band on holiday with you — this exercise still works without.

SUNBURN SQUATS

HOW TO DO IT: Place a loop band around your ankles. Stand straight with your core engaged and feet shoulder-width apart. Keeping your chest up, your abs pulled tight and your weight in your heels, drop your butt back into a squat.

Keeping your butt low, take a controlled step out to the side, feeling the resistance in the band the entire time.

Step the same foot back in, but don't let the band snap back in — move with control. Keep resistance on the band all the way through. Repeat these side steps with this leg for 30 seconds. Then swap legs. Feel the burn! **{30 seconds each leg, then skip for 30 seconds}**

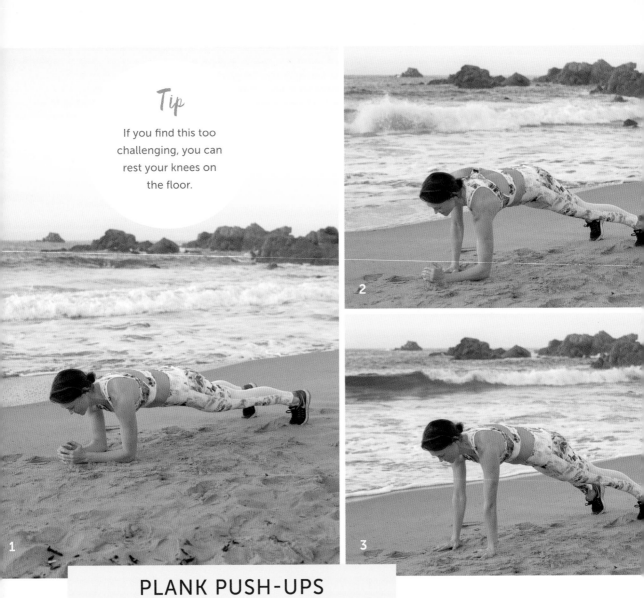

Tip

If you find this too challenging, you can rest your knees on the floor.

PLANK PUSH-UPS

HOW TO DO IT: Start in plank position with your elbows below your shoulders and your body in a straight line from your head to your heels. Engage your core.

One arm at a time, push yourself up into a high plank position.

Lower yourself, one arm at a time, back into the plank position. This is one rep of the plank-up. In your next rep, start by pushing up with the other arm. Keep alternating.

{30 seconds total, then skip for 30 seconds}

ACTIVE

TUMMY TIGHTENER

HOW TO DO IT: Lie on your back. Lift your legs, with your knees bent, into a tabletop position, shin parallel to the floor, knees above hips. Place your hands on your thighs. Press your lower back firmly into the floor, tightening your abs. Press your hands into your thighs as hard as you can. From the picture, this might look like a static exercise but trust me, you'll feel it! Hold firm for 30 seconds. **{30 seconds total, then return to the start of the workout for round two}**

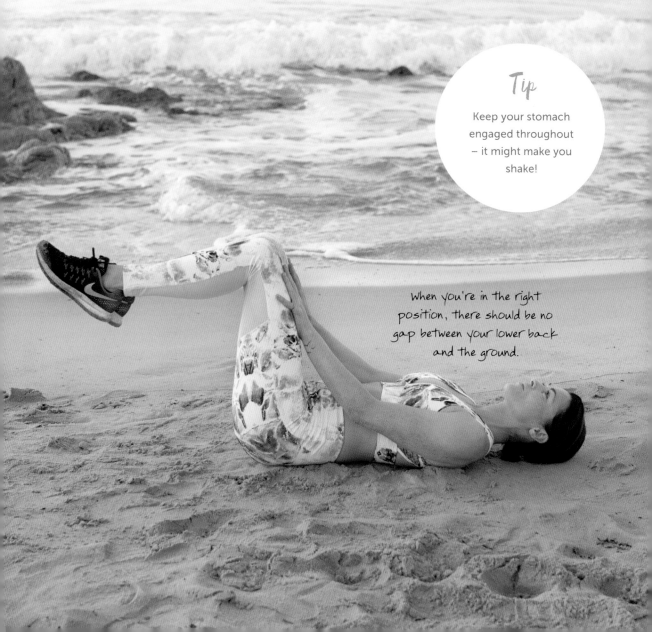

Tip

Keep your stomach engaged throughout – it might make you shake!

When you're in the right position, there should be no gap between your lower back and the ground.

KICK IT WORKOUT

A holiday is the perfect time to try something new, so this workout is all about kick boxing. I have a black belt in kick boxing and love incorporating it into my workouts. This is high energy, works every muscle, helps with balance and needs no equipment. Most important though, it's fun – just what you need on holiday. | **10 MINUTES (2 X 5 MINUTES)**

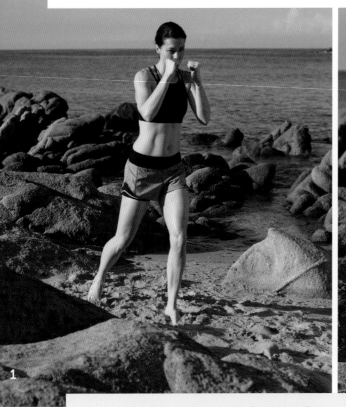

1

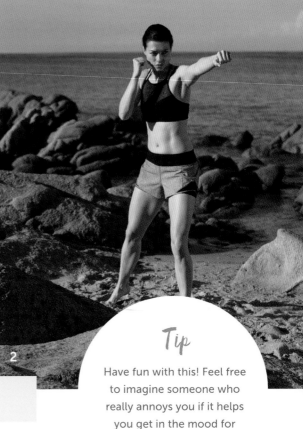

2

SHADOW BOXING

Tip

Have fun with this! Feel free to imagine someone who really annoys you if it helps you get in the mood for throwing a few punches!

HOW TO DO IT: Stand with one leg slightly forward and bring your fists upwards towards your chin into a fighting stance. Punch into the air with alternate arms. Be playful – don't become static, keep moving! Let your weight move, let your feet move, and really go for it. Keep going for 30 seconds. **{30 seconds total}**

ACTIVE

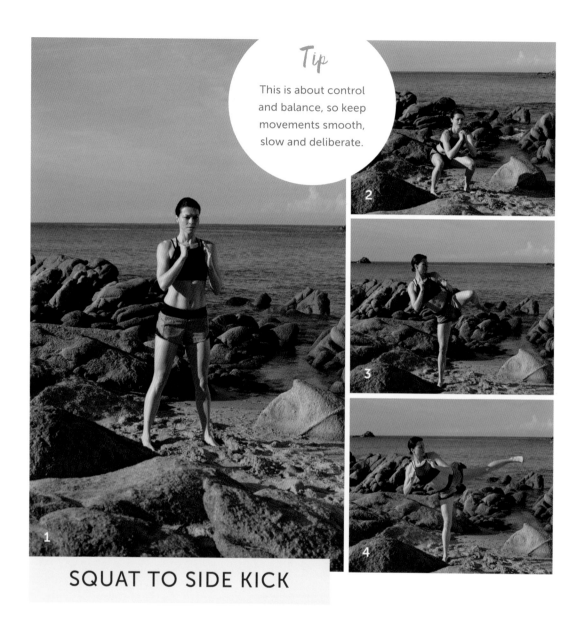

Tip

This is about control and balance, so keep movements smooth, slow and deliberate.

SQUAT TO SIDE KICK

HOW TO DO IT: Stand tall with your feet shoulder-width apart. Bend your knees and come into a squat position. Stand straight back up. Lean your weight onto your right foot and lift your left leg off the ground, bringing it up and out to the side with your knee bent and foot flexed. With control, straighten your leg into a full side kick. Bend your knee again, then lower the leg and return to a squat. Repeat for 30 seconds, then do the other side. **{30 seconds each leg}**

PLANK PUNCH

HOW TO DO IT: Start in a low plank position, with forearms resting on the ground and elbows under shoulders. Your feet should be shoulder-width apart. Lift your left arm and punch it forward, then place it back on the floor and repeat with the other arm. Keep repeating, alternating from side to side, for 30 seconds. **{30 seconds total}**

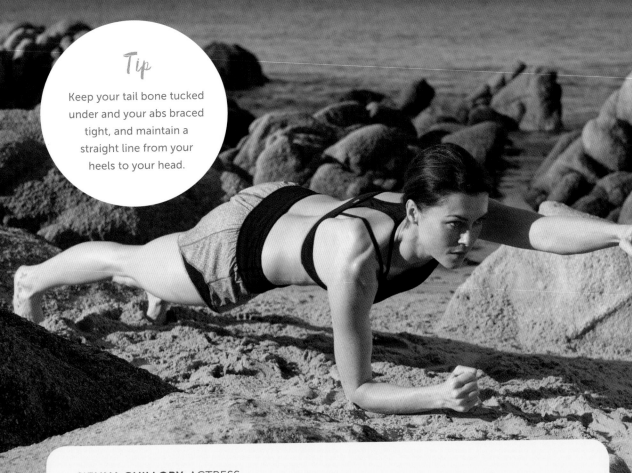

Tip

Keep your tail bone tucked under and your abs braced tight, and maintain a straight line from your heels to your head.

SIENNA GUILLORY, ACTRESS

'Kickboxing is one of the few exercises I genuinely enjoy doing, it's one of those things where technique is everything. Holly breaks down seriously impressive choreography into simple elements so that when I show up on a film set I have the confidence to style it out! I feel really proud to be able to perform my own stunts, and there's something balletic yet explosive about kickboxing that gives me real joy. The way it lengthens and tones my legs, bum and waist is kind of addictive too.'

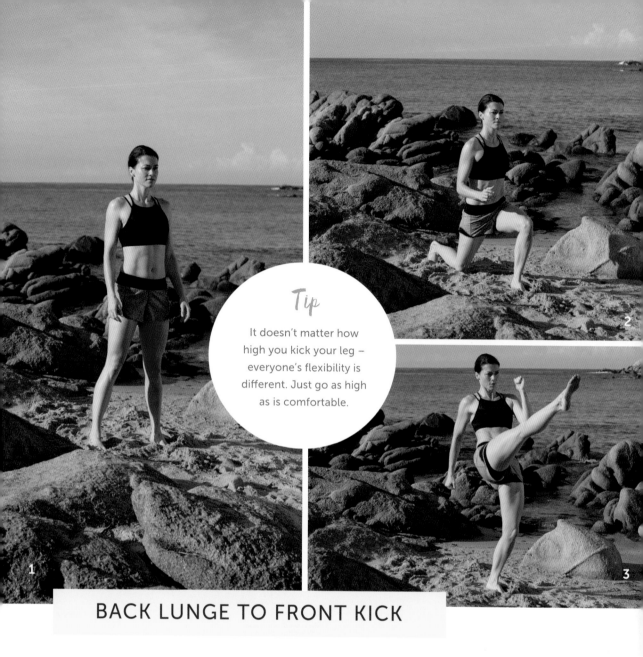

1

2

3

BACK LUNGE TO FRONT KICK

HOW TO DO IT: Stand tall with your feet shoulder-width apart. Take a big step back with your right leg into a back lunge, bending both knees to 90 degrees. With a big push off the foot, bring your right leg forwards and up into a front kick in one movement. Move straight back into the backward lunge and repeat for 30 seconds, then swap to the other leg and repeat for another 30 seconds. **{30 seconds each leg}**

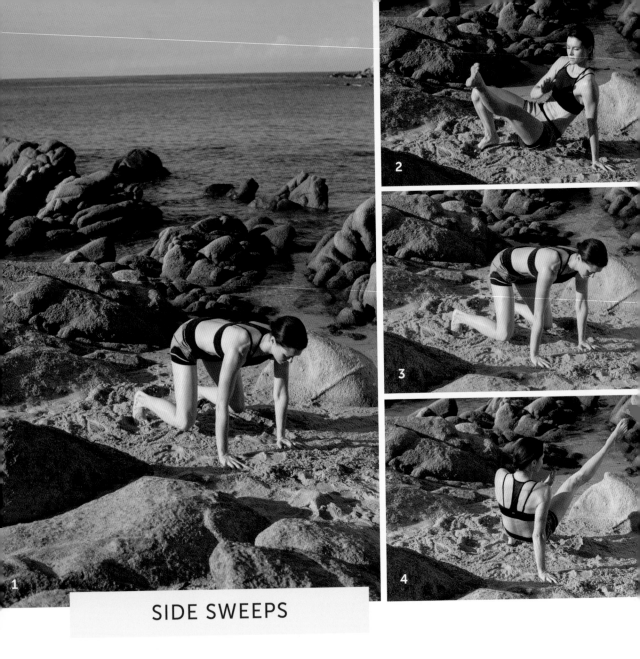

SIDE SWEEPS

HOW TO DO IT: Start on all fours. Tuck your toes under and bring your knees off the floor. Lift your left leg and right arm and twist to the right until your torso is facing upwards and your left butt cheek is almost touching the floor – but don't let it touch! Twist back to the previous position and repeat on the other side. Repeat for 30 seconds, alternating sides. **{30 seconds total}**

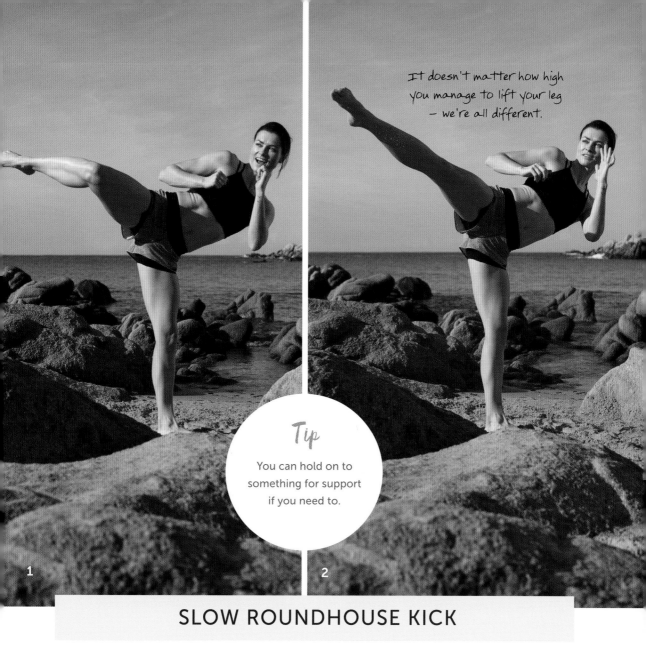

It doesn't matter how high you manage to lift your leg — we're all different.

Tip

You can hold on to something for support if you need to.

1

2

SLOW ROUNDHOUSE KICK

HOW TO DO IT: Stand tall with your feet shoulder-width apart and your fists raised. Lean your weight to your left and lift your right leg to balance with your right knee bent. Extend your right leg out so it's completely straight. Without lowering your foot to the ground, keep bending and extending the leg. Repeat for 30 seconds, then swap legs and do the same on the other side. **{30 seconds on each side}**

YOUR HOLIDAY DIET

Lots of my clients tell me that they struggle to eat well when they're away and ask for my advice, and so I tell them this. Whether you're on holiday or at home, forget rules, fads, calories and fat content and just eat delicious, nutritionally balanced, locally sourced foods with as many natural flavours (i.e. herbs and spices) and vegetables as possible. You're on holiday, though, so it's fine to treat yourself. Choose your daily indulgence and make it part of your holiday experience. You'll enjoy it more this way then overdoing it at every meal.

Here's a quick guide to the healthiest choices for just a few different destinations...

IF YOU'RE IN GREECE – take advantage of all the olives, Greek salads, fresh bread, local seafood and grilled chicken or vegetable kebabs.

IF YOU'RE IN SPAIN – tuck into stuffed peppers, paella, Spanish omelettes, fresh calamari and all the wonderful seafood.

IF YOU'RE IN FRANCE – the French tend to cook locally and seasonally and buy a lot of their food fresh from local markets. Different towns and cities enjoy different meals, but fresh fish, salads and mussels with crusty bread are always a good bet.

IF YOU'RE IN ITALY – avoid the creamy pasta dishes and opt for the tomato-based ones instead with green salads, olives and fresh bread.

IF YOU'RE IN THE UK – if you holiday on the UK coast, rather than just eating fish and chips, try the local seafood, which is some of the best around.

IF YOU'RE IN THE USA – watch your portion sizes and order a starter for your main and share sides. A chicken or vegetable burrito is a good choice, or grilled shrimp with salad.

IF YOU'RE IN THAILAND – it's easy to eat healthily here because their diet is naturally low in saturated fat and portions tend to be on the smaller side. You can enjoy seafood or chicken, which is often cooked in an abundance of fresh, local herbs and spices.

IF YOU'RE IN AUSTRALIA – another country where it's easy to be healthy; they serve lots of fresh fish, steaks, seafood and salad.

And remember, if you're eating out – don't devour the whole bread basket! If you're really hungry when you sit down, order a few salads or healthy salads to snack on.

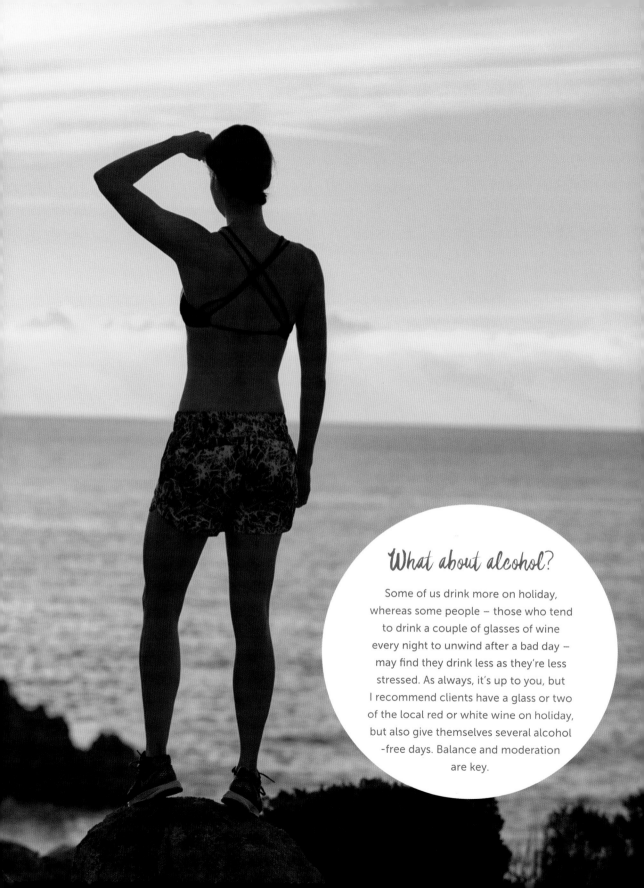

What about alcohol?

Some of us drink more on holiday, whereas some people – those who tend to drink a couple of glasses of wine every night to unwind after a bad day – may find they drink less as they're less stressed. As always, it's up to you, but I recommend clients have a glass or two of the local red or white wine on holiday, but also give themselves several alcohol-free days. Balance and moderation are key.

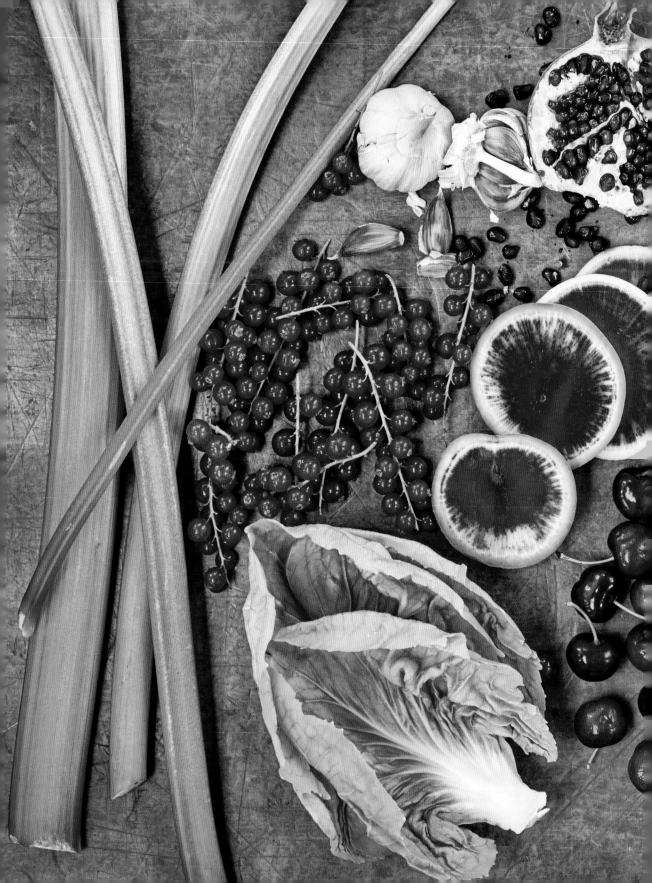

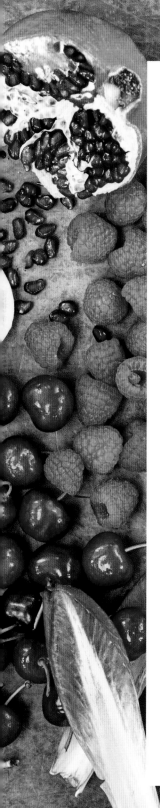

CHAPTER 7

A Word on Diet

There is no getting around the fact that, for a truly healthy lifestyle, exercise goes hand in hand with good eating. You simply won't feel as good as you'd like to if you do one without the other. If you eat well but live a fairly sedentary life, you'll never feel as fit, healthy and energised as you could. Similarly, if you go to the gym three times a week but eat junk food a lot, you'll always feel sluggish and heavy. Remember, you can't out-train a bad diet. However, the good news is that, when you start exercising regularly, you immediately find that you want to eat better too, especially so that all that good work doesn't go to waste.

For me, the key to eating well is actually very simple and involves what we've known for years. Essentially, the majority of our meals should be made up from a balance of fresh, seasonal and ideally organic vegetables, well-sourced grains, like wholegrain rice, quinoa and oats, and lean meat, chicken and fish. Personally, I was brought up as a vegetarian and it's how I enjoy eating. However, I know it's not for everyone and I certainly don't tell clients not to eat meat (page 137).

We also need a little healthy fat, like oils (olive oil and coconut oil are my favourites), oily fish, avocados, nuts and seeds, and plenty of water. But I also believe that everything should be in moderation, and I don't see a couple of glasses of wine or some chocolate as a treat. These can also be part of a healthy, balanced diet and should be guilt-free, if they're enjoyed in moderation.

I tell clients to fuel their body like an engine – you want to be putting the good stuff in there. If you wake up and have a really good, energising, nourishing, nutritious breakfast, you'll feel great for the day ahead. If you eat junk, on the other hand, you'll feel hungry and tired, you'll crave sugar and you'll feel sluggish and get ill more often.

But just as with exercise, I don't think it's helpful to see a healthy diet as a huge, overwhelming obstacle to tackle. Clients often tell me how, when they start a new diet, they cut out all their favourite treats, they tell themselves they're never going to drink again and they start reducing their portion sizes so they're having tiny bowls of porridge for breakfast or just salads for lunch. Predictably, they very quickly become bored with this way of eating, feel extremely hungry and revert to their old ways.

It's a good idea to start small. First look at the food that you eat regularly and enjoy and tweak this. Make a few healthy additions and remove anything that is sabotaging your good work, but stick with foods that you know and love and want to eat. This keeps things simple and won't make you feel you're 'on a diet' at all. And as I've said in Chapter 1 about the ebbs and flows of exercise, the same applies to food. If you manage to eat

well for a few days and then dive into a bar of chocolate, don't worry about it. Let it pass and go back to better habits the next day. In the checklist below I've shared my three guiding principles. It's a great place to start.

MY HEALTHY-EATING CHECKLIST

- Check food labels to make sure you're not eating lots of sugar without realising. 'Diet' foods are notorious for this, especially yogurts, cereals, and ready meals.
- Cook from scratch so you know exactly what's going into your body.
- You don't need to become teetotal, but don't drink two glasses of wine every single night either, purely out of habit. Find other ways to relax in the evening, like reading a good book, going to the gym or having a nice bath. Overdoing it on the wine can leave you feeling sluggish next day, making you less likely to work out and more likely to reach for less healthy foods.

keep a food diary

A food diary can be a massive eye opener as people assume they're eating OK but, when they see it written down, they realise their portions are too big or they're having something sweet after every meal, or snacking on the wrong things in between meals and drinking wine every night. We all have a weak spot – sometimes more than one – and a food diary is a good way of highlighting what that is. And once you know, you can take steps to address it.

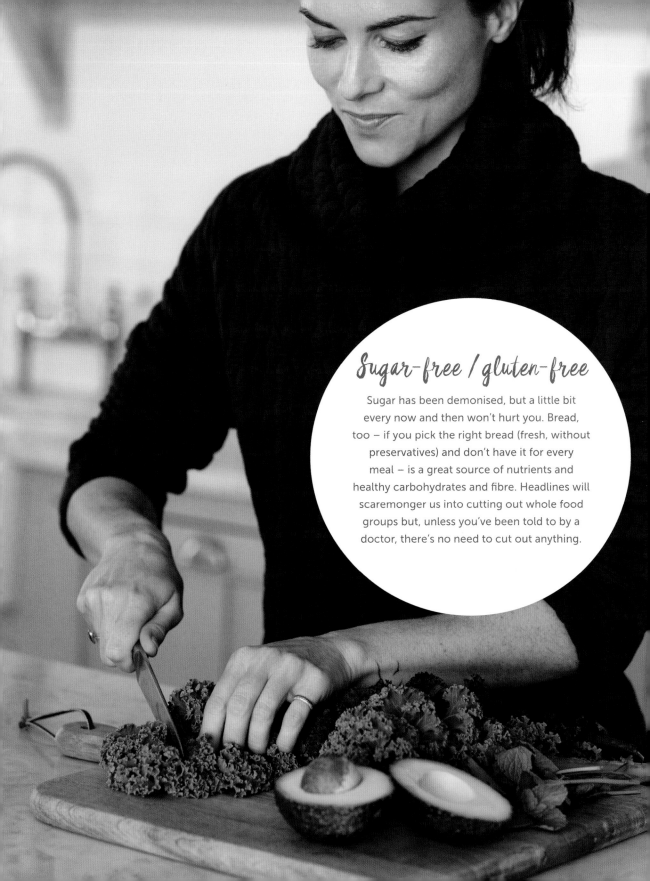

Sugar-free / gluten-free

Sugar has been demonised, but a little bit every now and then won't hurt you. Bread, too – if you pick the right bread (fresh, without preservatives) and don't have it for every meal – is a great source of nutrients and healthy carbohydrates and fibre. Headlines will scaremonger us into cutting out whole food groups but, unless you've been told to by a doctor, there's no need to cut out anything.

WHAT I EAT IN A DAY

Clients often ask me what I eat, so here goes (and for more inspiration, head to pages 145–67, where you'll find lots of my favourite recipes).

BREAKFAST

2 scrambled or poached eggs on a slice of sourdough or rye toast with ½ avocado on the side.

OR My own nutty granola mix that I make myself – a small handful or tablespoon of goji berries, toasted coconut flakes, cocoa nibs, pumpkin seeds and walnuts mixed in a bowl. I then serve it with a good dollop of organic goat's yogurt or oat milk and add a handful of seasonal berries on top (raspberries, blueberries or blackberries are my favourite).

OR A smoothie – if I'm rushing out the door, I'll throw some frozen berries, ½ banana, ¼ avocado, a handful of spinach, some almond, coconut or oat milk in my blender and have it on the go.

LUNCH

A homemade salad: If I'm at home, I'll make a salad that contains quinoa, lentils or beans, cottage cheese or hummus, lots of green vegetables like rocket or roasted kale, then a little fat such as olive oil or ½ avocado. Your lunch must contain some protein and a little good fat, otherwise you'll be hungry all afternoon.

OR Soup: try my carrot and lentil soup on page 153.

DINNER

Again, I often make a salad – a large handful of spinach leaves, a small handful of walnuts, 5–6 baby tomatoes roasted with garlic, ½ avocado, some fermented cabbage, a spoonful of hummus and 1–2 buckwheat crackers. This is one of my favourites, but you can mix and match similar ingredients to make your own version. I love a combination of different textures and flavours when it comes to food – a bit of crunch, something nutty or creamy, something sweet and so on.

In the winter, I love making a hearty stew and simply throw my favourite vegetables into a casserole dish with some kidney beans and some vegetable stock.

Spiralised courgette with coconut oil and pesto – this is my favourite quick supper. I'll spiralise a few courgettes and lightly fry them for a minute or so in coconut oil and then stir through some pesto.

Holly's favourite snacks

- A few celery sticks with hummus
- A small handful of nuts and toasted seeds
- A hard-boiled egg
- A homemade energy ball (page 163)
- ½ avocado on a buckwheat cracker
- 2 squares of 90 per cent dark chocolate

SNACKING

Some experts are against snacking as they think it raises blood-sugar levels and keeps them elevated throughout the day, which can lead to insulin resistance and weight gain. But I believe everybody is different. It's good to have three healthy, nourishing meals a day, so aim for that. However, if you need to snack in between, then go ahead. Don't do it because you're bored, and try to snack on the right things (see left). I have clients who leave work at 6 and don't get home until 7 or 8pm. If they've had lunch at 1pm, they need a snack to keep going until dinner time. So like everything else, do what's right for you.

VEGETARIANISM

I was raised a vegetarian, so I've never had any meat or fish in my diet. When I was growing up, I was always given the choice to eat meat or fish if I wanted to, but I never felt I was missing out and so never did.

As a vegetarian, I find that there is an abundance of delicious, healthy food choices – now more so than ever – and I'm always keen to promote it. However, I'd never tell any of my clients (or friends) to give up meat. Many of them enjoy eating it and I'm always happy to give them recipe and meal ideas that include meat and fish, as I do throughout this book. The thing I do recommend, though, is to be smarter about meat (and dairy too). My father is a very ethical man and he was always questioning where his food came from and how it was produced and, for that reason, I recommend clients buy organic meat and dairy. Animals reared for meat and dairy are often given antibiotics and hormones to make them bigger or to produce more milk, which can have a negative impact on our health. I'm not a vegan and I will have egg and a little bit of organic cheese, but if I'm having dairy, it has to be organic. If you can't afford to buy organic meat, then perhaps buy a little less of it and I always tell clients that, if they eat red meat, they should limit it to once a week.

ZOE, 41, INTERIORS JOURNALIST AND MUM OF THREE

'I've always been reasonably fit but after the birth of my third child at the age of 35 I was exhausted and I felt that I'd hit a road block.

'Holly started me training at different times of day, such as at 6.45am when the kids were still in bed, or after school drop-off, or sometimes mid-morning when coffee was already in my system. And she'd make me plan my lunch while we were running so I didn't lose focus and eat the wrong food post-workout.

'I was also skipping breakfast to do the school run, so Holly got me into breakfast smoothies.

'Holly made me keep a food diary to pinpoint where I was going wrong. I knew I had a tendency to snack mindlessly after dinner when I wasn't hungry, but seeing it all written down helped me take control of it. After just a couple of months, I did look better. But it's more than just that – I feel healthier, stronger and much happier too.'

Meat-free Mondays, 'Flexitarianism' (i.e. a flexible vegetarian who sometimes eats meat) and part-time vegetarianism are on the rise and, rather than seeing it as a fad, I see it as a really positive movement and shows people questioning where their food is coming from and taking steps to improve their health. Being a part-time vegetarian is very easy to achieve and research from Mintel in 2017 found that, in the last few years, almost half of British people have reduced their meat intake or are considering doing so, primarily for health reasons. Statistics from The Vegan Society also now record that there are over half a million vegans in the UK.

When I was growing up, vegetarianism was nowhere near as popular as it is today and my school and schoolfriends' parents were always a bit stumped as to what food to give me. Typically, they gave me pasta and, when I went to restaurants, the only choices on the menu for me were pasta, risotto or some sort of processed meat substitute, like vegetarian sausages or pie. Thankfully, things have changed for the better and now plants have taken centre stage on our plates. Foods like kale have become the new superfoods. There are some fantastic vegetarian restaurants around and even regular restaurants offer great meat-free meals that aren't necessarily even labelled 'vegetarian'.

In terms of health, there are a few things you need to consider when you're a vegetarian. Firstly, you must replace your meat with protein. Some 'flexitarians', or flexible vegetarians, may eat fish, and that's their source of protein. However, if you're fully vegetarian, you can get your protein from things like lentils, pulses and beans, soya and tofu, yogurt, nuts, nut milks and eggs.

It's also important to supplement properly. I take vitamin B12 because meat is its best source and, as a vegetarian, I have to keep an eye on my levels. B12 is a water-soluble vitamin that keeps your red blood cells healthy and, if you're deficient, you can suffer from low energy levels. Non-meat foods like walnuts contain B12, but meat is the best source.

A WORD ON SUPPLEMENTS

Here is a list of the supplements that I personally take. However, I'm not suggesting that you take the exact same combination because it's impossible for me to give you advice when I don't know you or your lifestyle and medical history. Everybody's needs are very specific and individual so it's best to see a qualified nutritionist or nutritional therapist who can provide you with the best information.

Vitamin D: Most British people are vitamin D-deficient because the sun is the best source of vitamin D and we simply don't get enough of it in this country. This important vitamin is responsible for calcium absorption, so it's vital for healthy bones and teeth, and low levels have even been linked to certain cancers and diabetes. I love Betteryou Vitamin D and have taken it for years.

Zinc: I take this to strengthen my digestive and immune systems and to improve my memory.

Turmeric: This is a fantastic natural anti-inflammatory that can help ward off a whole host of ills, including heart disease and diabetes.

A BALANCED DIET

As I said at the beginning of the chapter, the truth is that exercise and a healthy diet are two sides of the same coin. I also outlined what I believe represents a healthy way to eat – a balanced diet made up of fresh, seasonal, ideally organic vegetables, well-sourced lentils, pulses, beans and grains, well-sourced organic dairy and a little healthy fat, like oils (olive oil and coconut oil), avocados, nuts and seeds, and plenty of water. If you eat meat, you should also include lean meat, such as chicken, and oily fish. However, let's break it down and take a closer look at the building blocks of a healthy diet that will fully complement your physical workouts.

WHAT'S THE DEAL WITH PROTEIN?

Protein is an essential component in our diet. Why? Because organs, tissues, muscles and hormones are all made up of proteins. In fact, every cell in the body contains proteins and so, unless they're continuously replenished through our diet, our bodies struggle to develop, grow and function properly. If we don't consume enough, our muscles and bones waste away, we find it hard to concentrate and experience 'brain fog', our metabolism becomes sluggish, our blood-sugar levels unstable and the list goes on. A lack of protein in the diet also contributes to weight gain as it's the protein in a meal that produces a sense of feeling 'full' and therefore prevents us overeating and oversnacking. As I said earlier in the chapter, try to include a little protein with every meal that you eat as this will keep your energy levels up, ward off cravings and blood-sugar highs and lows and make it much much easier for you to keep to a healthy diet.

HOW MUCH PROTEIN DO YOU ACTUALLY NEED?

Well, an easy way to answer this is to make sure you include protein with all your meals and snacks. Don't have carbohydrate-only meals, like bowls of pasta with a sauce and little in the way of protein, for example.

WHERE CAN YOU FIND GOOD PROTEIN?

Here's a list of foods that are a good source of protein and should be included in your meals and snacks.

- Organic chicken
- Well-sourced fish
- Organic eggs
- Beans
- Nuts
- Nut milks (for example almond, coconut or hemp milk, which are fairly good sources of protein. Non-dairy milks like oat milk are carbohydrate-based and don't contain as much protein)
- Organic cheese (most kinds, but again steer clear of the processed kinds)

WHAT ABOUT PROTEIN POWDERS AND SUPPLEMENTS?

There are lots of these around nowadays and, while some can be fantastically healthy, others contain sweeteners and processed ingredients. The best advice, as with everything, is do your research and start by reading the labels on the packet.

Post-work out food

It's important to eat protein after exercise, especially after strength training so that your muscles repair and grow back stronger. For a quick protein fix post-workout, try a protein shake or an omelette. If you have a bit more time, my quinoa bowl on page 148 is a great protein source. Or, if you eat fish, try the salmon dish on page 152.

I take Sun Warrior Classic Plus Organic protein powder because it's natural and a really well-sourced plant-based powder, plus it doesn't contain any dairy (lots of them do). I don't take it every day, but I do take it in a smoothie if I'm short on time before or after a workout.

Similarly, there are lots of so-called 'super green powders' around too. I think some of them are great, especially if you're not going to eat many greens in your diet on a given day and feel like topping up. However, some of them can be very expensive and I don't like the idea of health being in some way elitist,

expensive or complicated. If you're eating something dark green and leafy every day, like broccoli, kale, asparagus or spinach (which you should be, so please do!), then I see no reason why you need to buy an expensive green powder on top of this. Unless you have the money and you want to, of course!

WHAT'S THE DEAL WITH CARBOHYDRATES?

Carbs have been getting a bad rap for a while now. However, they shouldn't be neglected as the body needs them to make glucose, its main source of energy. They also provide many key nutrients and we need them to function well. However, carbs come in many different shapes and sizes and what's important is to distinguish the good from the bad and to choose them wisely. The best carbs are fibre-rich vegetables, fruits and wholegrains as it's the fibre that slows down the release of energy and provides the nutrients too. Bad carbs, which often deserve their bad rap, are those that have been processed and where the fibre has been stripped and sugar added (e.g. white pasta, white bread, etc).

PRE-WORKOUT FOODS?

A banana or a handful of nuts will give you a quick boost before you work out. For an endurance-based exercise, such as a long run, a bowl of porridge with almond butter and banana will keep you going. However, be careful of eating too close to a workout – it could give you a stitch or make you feel sick.

WHAT'S THE DEAL WITH FAT?

The word 'fat' can be rather off-putting. However, the key thing to remember is that fat doesn't make us fat. In fact, the opposite is the case as, like protein, it provides us with that sensation of a full stomach and so banishes cravings and the temptation to overeat and oversnack, which are the main culprits when it comes to weight gain. Fat is also one of our best sources of energy. For every gram of fat that you eat, you get 9 calories of fuel for your body, which is more than double that provided by carbs and protein, which both deliver 4 calories per gram. And without fat in our diets, we would all be deficient in essential nutrients, as vitamins A, E and K are all fat-soluble.

The key thing to keep in mind, however, is that not all fats are created equal and, as with carbs, you have to know the good from the bad. While eggs, avocados, full-fat cheese, milk and butter, oily fish, nuts, seeds and vegetable oils are all healthy fats, chips, doughnuts and other processed foods are not. In particular, be wary of any foods that are labelled 'low-fat' as these often come laden with sweeteners, preservatives and artificial flavours. The source of your fat should therefore always be natural and I recommend a balance, too, so it's not all dairy-based but also derived from vegetables, nuts and seeds.

FERMENTED FOODS

In my food diary, you may have spotted that I listed fermented cabbage as a favourite ingredient. I think it's delicious and also love the fact that it comes with a whole host of health benefits. Many of these come from the fermenting process as it produces all kinds of beneficial probiotics (bacteria) that help you maintain healthy cognitive, immune and digestive systems. You only need to eat a small amount daily to reap the rewards, so I often add a spoonful of sauerkraut to salads. However, you can experiment with different types of fermented foods, such as kefir (cultured dairy), kimchi (a Korean classic) or any kind of fermented fruit, grain or vegetable to find your own preference.

HYDRATION

I couldn't have a chapter on good eating without mentioning good drinking. Drinking enough water is crucial for every single cell and every single function in the body, yet so many of us let proper hydration slip down our to-do list and only take a sip of water when we're already thirsty (and therefore already dehydrated). Or worse, we drink sugary drinks to quench our thirst. So my hydration rules are simple: drink often throughout the day and drink mainly water. If you drink alcohol or a lot of caffeinated drinks, then you need even more water to counter the effects, so tea, coffee, alcohol and sugary drinks simply don't count (but herbal teas do).

There's no hard and fast rule on how much water you should be drinking, so don't get too caught up in trying to keep track of exactly how many glasses or litres of water you have a day. Instead of keeping count, do the following:

- Drink a glass of water (not tea) when you wake up and before you have breakfast or your first coffee of the day.

- Drink a glass of water 30 minutes before each meal and snack.
- Have a glass of water on your desk at work and sip it regularly.
- If you're not desk-based during the day, have a refillable water bottle with you at all times and refill it regularly.
- Drink a glass of water after every caffeinated drink.
- Eat water-rich foods like cucumber, celery, spinach and melon (watermelon is the best water source), and other fruits and vegetables.

ARE YOU DRINKING ENOUGH?

- Check your urine – it should be the colour of pale straw. If it's darker, drink more water!
- Do you get frequent headaches or brain fog, especially in the afternoons? Ditch the headache pills and simply drink more water!
- Are you often hungry? Mild dehydration can often be mistaken for hunger or lead to sugar cravings. So before you reach for a snack, try drinking a glass of water.
- Does your mouth often feel dry or do you worry you have bad breath? A dry mouth from dehydration can lead to a build up of bacteria in the mouth, which can cause bad breath. The solution? You guessed it – drink a glass of water.

Lastly, I'm often asked what I think about coconut water and I think it makes a very good sports drink. So if you're doing a lot of running or exercise, then it's fine. It contains more potassium that regular sports drinks and more natural sources of sodium, so it's much better for you than some of the big name sports drinks out there. But if you're not exercising a lot, be careful with it because it's very sweet. When it comes to hydration, water is the best.

FOODS THAT MAKE YOU FLEXIBLE

With all the exercise that you're doing, it's obviously important to keep your joints nice and flexible to guard against aches and injury. Luckily, there are certain foods that can help a lot with reducing inflammation and stiffness, so include them in your diet:

- Brazil nuts
- Peppers
- Broccoli
- Cauliflower
- Onions
- Leeks
- Butternut squash
- Citrus fruits (oranges, kiwis, grapefruit, lemons, limes, etc.)
- Cherries
- Green tea

The following foods, however, have been shown to increase inflammation, so try to limit them:

- Alcohol
- Sugar
- Processed foods

RECIPES

On the following pages I've shared a few of my favourite recipes. Although I'm a vegetarian, I've suggested a couple of options with fish, or you can play around and add chicken if you like.

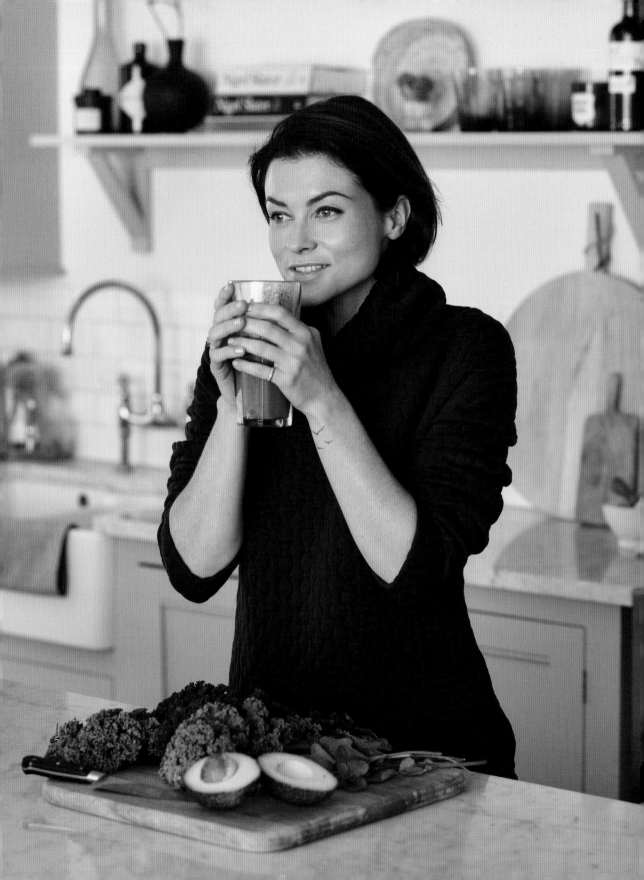

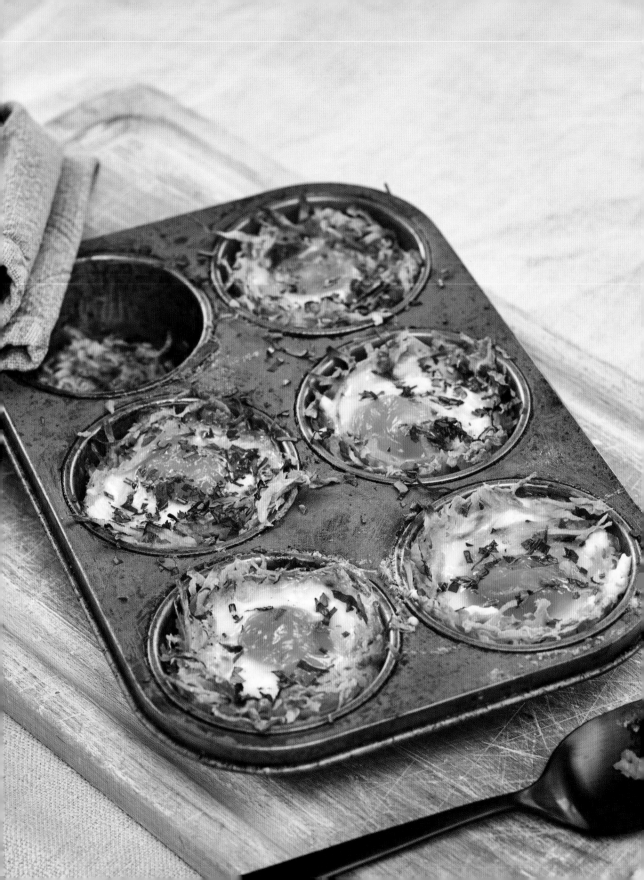

Egg Muddle

BEST FOR: Lazy weekend breakfasts
MAKES: 6

coconut oil, for greasing

½ sweet potato, peeled and grated

100g/¾ cup organic feta cheese

6 eggs

1 tablespoon of your favourite chopped herbs, such as basil, coriander or parsley

sea salt and freshly ground black pepper, to taste

Preheat the oven to 180°C/350°F/gas mark 4. Grease the bottoms and sides of a 6-hole muffin tin with a little coconut oil.

Divide the sweet potato between the moulds and press down to form a thin nest in each.

Crumble a small amount of feta on top, then crack one egg into each mould (ensuring the yolk stays intact). Sprinkle with herbs and season with salt and pepper.

Cook for 15 minutes, or until the egg is cooked through, then carefully turn out onto plates and serve immediately, allowing 1–2 per serving.

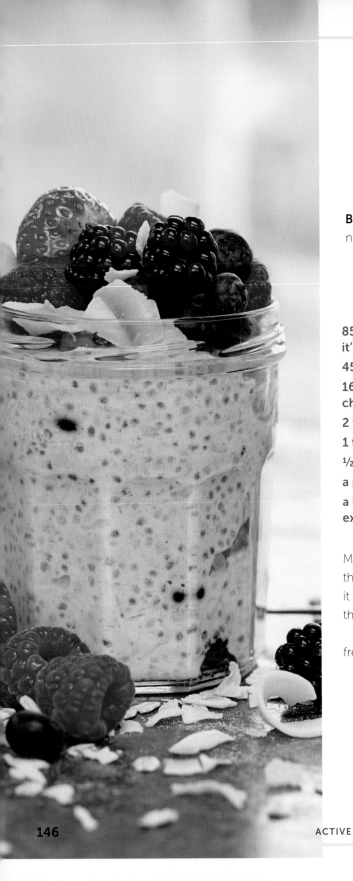

Overnight oats

BEST FOR: A busy week. You can prep it the night before and grab it on your way out the door to work.

SERVES: 1

85g (⅓ cup) plain Greek yogurt (make sure it's not low fat)

45g (½ cup) rolled oats

160ml (¾ cup) unsweetened milk of your choice (I use almond)

2 tablespoons toasted flaked coconut

1 tablespoon chia seeds

½ teaspoon vanilla extract

a pinch of sea salt

a handful of your favourite berries, plus extra to serve

Mix all the ingredients together in a bowl, then spoon into a glass jar and seal or cover it with clingfilm. Leave to soak overnight in the fridge.

In the morning, stir and serve with extra fresh berries.

ACTIVE

Spinach and cheese frittatas

BEST FOR: A late weekend breakfast, perhaps when you have friends round. These can be stored in the fridge for a day or two and taste great eaten cold with salad for a quick lunch.

MAKES: 12

coconut oil, for greasing

6 large eggs

285ml (1¼ cups) milk

sea salt and freshly ground black pepper, to taste

220g (2 cups) soft goat's cheese, crumbled

½ red pepper

a handful of spinach leaves, chopped

Preheat the oven to 180°C/350°F/gas mark 4 and grease the bottoms and sides of a 12-hole muffin tin.

In a bowl, beat the eggs and milk with a pinch of salt and black pepper, then stir in the cheese, red pepper and spinach.

Divide the mixture between the moulds and bake for 20 minutes, or until the egg mixture is set.

Cool slightly, then carefully tip out onto plates and serve warm, allowing 2 per serving.

Tip

These can be kept in the fridge for up to three days.

Quinoa breakfast bowl

BEST FOR: This is a great protein-packed breakfast to have before or after a morning workout. It also makes a great lunch if you have any left over.

SERVES: 2

100g (½ cup) quinoa

splash of white wine vinegar

4 eggs

a handful of sunflower seeds

a handful of your favourite herbs (such as parsley, basil, coriander and mint), chopped

a handful of room temperature cherry tomatoes, halved

2 handfuls of spinach leaves

juice of 1 lemon

a drizzle of cold-pressed olive oil

sea salt and freshly ground black pepper, to taste

Cook the quinoa according to the packet instructions, then set aside to cool slightly.

Bring a pan of water to the boil, then reduce to a simmer. Add the vinegar, then crack in the eggs, one by one (don't crowd the pan). Poach the eggs for 3–4 minutes, then remove with a slotted spoon and drain on kitchen paper.

Meanwhile, toast the sunflower seeds for 2 minutes in a dry frying pan over a medium heat, until they smell nutty.

Place the quinoa in a mixing bowl and stir in the herbs. Add the tomatoes, seeds and spinach leaves, then toss everything in the lemon juice and olive oil and season with salt and pepper to taste.

Serve in bowls with the poached eggs arranged on top.

Tip

If you want a variation, you can swap the lemon juice and olive oil for my everyday salad dressing on page 159.

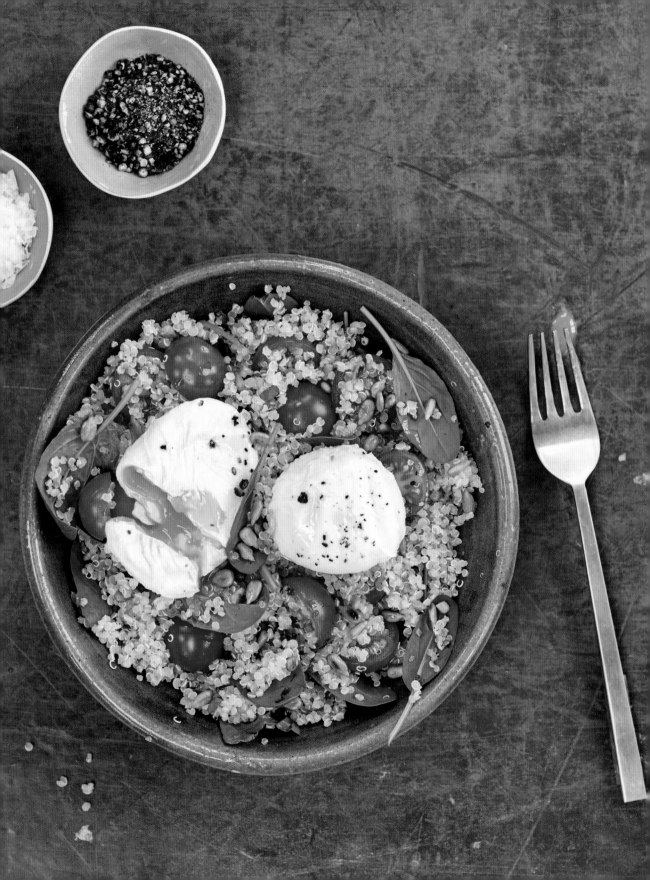

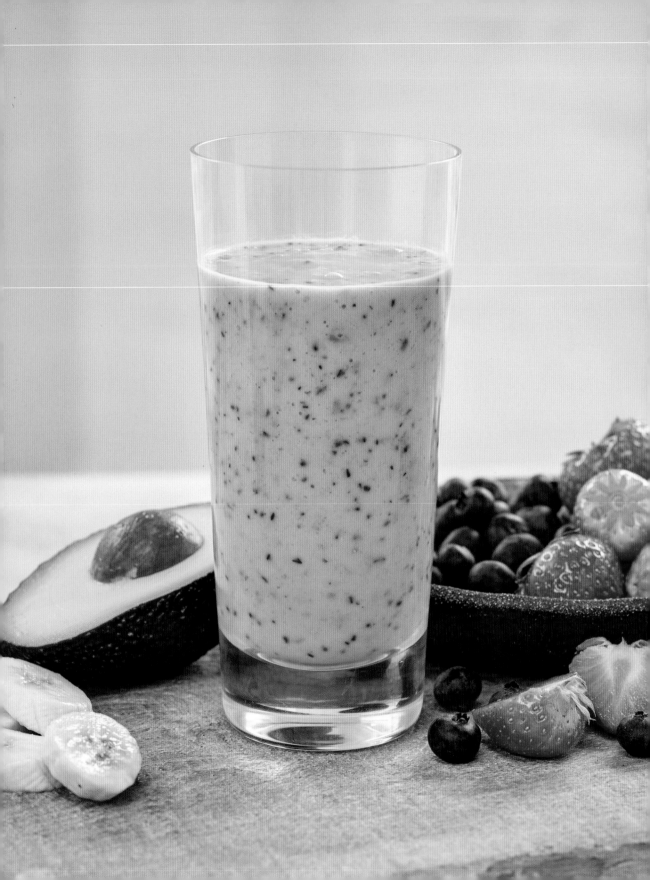

Avocado and berry smoothie

BEST FOR: A quick, light breakfast for people who don't really 'do' breakfast.

SERVES: 1

½ **banana**

¼ **avocado**

10 **blueberries**

8–10 **strawberries**

240ml (1 cup) **unsweetened almond, coconut or oat milk**

Place all the ingredients in a blender or food processer and blitz until smooth and creamy. If you like a thinner consistency, add more milk or a little water.

Tip

I like my smoothie thick and creamy and usually eat it from a bowl with a spoon. I find this makes me eat it more slowly and I enjoy it more.

Salmon with courgetti pesto

BEST FOR: This is a quick, easy, filling lunch that can be eaten hot or cold. I sometimes make my own pesto, but I also buy it too, so if you're short on time simply buy a good-quality organic one with as few ingredients as possible.

SERVES: 1

1 skinless salmon fillet
olive oil, for brushing
a squeeze of lemon juice
2 courgettes
a handful of rocket, to serve

FOR THE PESTO:
a handful of cashew nuts
a handful of sunflower seeds
a handful of spinach leaves
a handful of basil leaves
1 teaspoon olive oil
sea salt and freshly ground black pepper, to taste

Preheat the oven to 180°C/350°F/gas mark 4.

Place the salmon on a piece of tin foil and brush with a little olive oil. Season with salt and pepper and a squeeze of lemon. Wrap the foil loosely around the salmon to form a parcel. Place this on a baking tray and bake for 12–15 minutes until the salmon flakes easily with a fork.

Meanwhile, using a spiraliser, turn the courgettes into 'courgetti'. If you don't have a spiraliser, simply peel or julienne the courgettes into very thin strips, then set aside.

Place all the pesto ingredients in a food processor or blender and blitz to a pesto-like texture.

Stir the pesto into the courgetti until it's thoroughly coated, then gently heat in a frying pan for two minutes. Arrange on a plate with the rocket. Top with the cooked salmon and season with an extra grinding of black pepper.

Veggie tip

Swap the salmon for half a can of chickpeas —just add them to the pan at the same time as the courgetti.

Chickpea couscous with broccoli and feta

BEST FOR: This is great post-workout as it's packed full of protein.

SERVES: 4

175g (1 cup) couscous

1 broccoli crown, broken into small florets

½ red onion, finely chopped

1 carrot, peeled and grated

40g (¹/₃ cup) cashew nuts, chopped

2 tablespoons white wine vinegar

1½ tablespoons olive oil

1 teaspoon ground turmeric

1 teaspoon diced fresh ginger

a large pinch of sea salt

400g (15oz) can chickpeas, drained and rinsed

150g (1½ cups) feta cheese, crumbled

sea salt and freshly ground black pepper, to taste

Prepare the couscous according to the packet instructions and set aside.

Place the broccoli in a steamer and cook for 3 minutes until just tender.

Fluff up the couscous with a fork, then transfer it to a large bowl with the broccoli and add all the remaining ingredients, except the feta. Mix until well combined, season to taste, then sprinkle the feta over the top and serve.

Carrot and lentil soup

BEST FOR: This is a very quick, easy and warming meal to eat on the go, so perfect for when you're busy but need something nourishing.

SERVES: 2

2 teaspoons olive oil

1 red onion, chopped

2 carrots, peeled and chopped into small cubes

2–3 garlic cloves, crushed

85g (½ cup) lentils or quinoa

1 vegetable stock cube

sourdough or wholemeal roll, to serve (optional)

Heat the oil in a frying pan over a medium heat and gently fry the onion for 2 minutes until soft but not brown.

Add the carrots and garlic and cook for a further minute.

Add 1 litre boiling water, then stir in the lentils or quinoa and add the stock cube. Cover and cook on a medium heat for 10–15 minutes until the carrots are softened and the lentils are tender.

Remove from the heat and either serve immediately or wait for it to cool and then purée in a blender (if you prefer a smoother soup), then reheat. Serve with toasted and buttered sourdough or a crusty wholemeal roll, if you like.

Warm butter bean, pomegranate and halloumi salad

BEST FOR: You can play around with the ingredients in this salad and swap the halloumi for chicken, or try it with half chicken and half halloumi. Grilled salmon also works well.

SERVES: 1

1 tablespoon flaked almonds, toasted

1 teaspoon coconut oil

100g (3½oz) halloumi cheese, cut into thick slices

½ x 400g (15oz) can butter beans, drained

100g (¾ cup) green beans

100g (¾ cup) cherry tomatoes, halved

3 sun-dried tomatoes, roughly chopped (optional)

seeds of ½ pomegranate

juice and zest of ½ orange

a handful of rocket, roughly chopped

1 teaspoon olive oil

sea salt and freshly ground black pepper, to taste

Preheat the oven to 180°C/350°F/gas mark 4. Arrange the almonds on a baking tray and toast lightly in the oven for 4–5 minutes. Keep an eye on them to prevent them from burning.

Meanwhile, heat the coconut oil in a frying pan and gently fry the halloumi on both sides until golden.

Heat the butter beans and the green beans in a pan of boiling water for 2 minutes, then drain and pop in a large bowl.

Add all the remaining ingredients and toss to combine. Top with the halloumi, sprinkle with the toasted almonds and serve immediately.

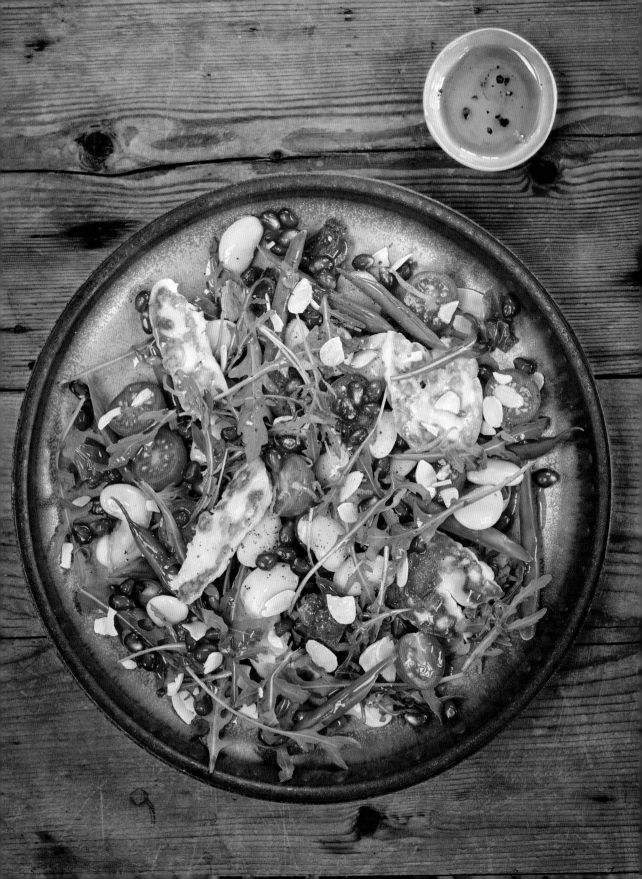

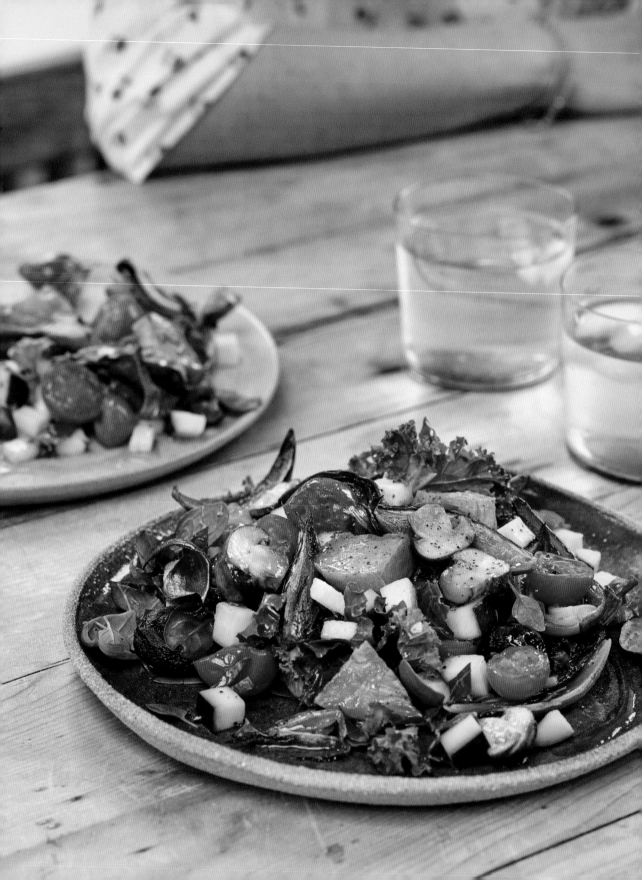

Roasted veggie salad

BEST FOR: This is an immunity-boosting powerhouse of a meal and perfect for the changing seasons when our immunity is low and we need a reboot.

SERVES: 2

FOR THE ROASTED VEGETABLES:

½ red onion, cut into wedges

½ small squash, cut into chunks

5 cherry tomatoes, halved

5–6 mushrooms

a drizzle of olive oil

sea salt and freshly ground black pepper, to taste

FOR THE SALAD:

a handful or coriander, chopped

a handful of basil leaves, chopped

a handful of kale, chopped

a handful of spinach leaves, chopped

1 courgette, diced

2–3 teaspoons olive oil

juice of ½ lemon

Preheat the oven to 180°C/350°F/gas mark 4.

Place the vegetables on a baking tray, drizzle with a little oil, season with salt and black pepper and bake for 20–25 minutes.

Meanwhile, in a large bowl, toss all the salad ingredients together. Season with salt and pepper.

Allow the vegetables to cool slightly, then add to the salad bowl and mix thoroughly. Season with salt and pepper and serve immediately.

Sweet potato, spinach and chickpea curry

BEST FOR: This is one of my favourite warming, comforting recipes when the days start to get darker or if I'm feeling run down or stressed. Add a little chicken if you like.

SERVES: 4

1 tablespoon coconut oil

1 large onion, chopped

2 garlic cloves, finely chopped

2.5cm (1in) piece of ginger, grated (you can leave the skin on)

1 teaspoon curry powder

1 cardamom pod

1 teaspoon ground turmeric

1 teaspoon chilli powder

1 teaspoon cumin

1 fresh red chilli, deseeded (unless you like curries very hot) and finely sliced

½ large pumpkin (or 2 sweet potatoes if pumpkins aren't in season or not easily available), peeled and cut into chunks

400g (15oz) can chickpeas, drained and rinsed

400ml (15oz) can coconut milk

200g (4 cups) baby leaf spinach

juice of 1 lime

a handful of fresh mint leaves, chopped

rice or quinoa, to serve (optional)

sea salt and freshly ground black pepper, to taste

Place the coconut oil in a large, heavy-based saucepan and gently fry the onion for 5 minutes until soft but not brown. Stir in the garlic and ginger and cook for a further 2-3 minutes.

Add the curry powder, cardamom, turmeric, chilli powder, cumin and fresh chilli, plus a splash of water. Season with salt and black pepper and cook, stirring, for 1 minute until the spices release their aromas.

Add the pumpkin or sweet potatoes and stir to coat in the spices.

Add the chickpeas and coconut milk and simmer for 20–30 minutes over a medium heat.

Add the spinach and stir in to wilt, then add the lime juice and scatter with the mint leaves.

Serve with rice or quinoa or enjoy just as it is, on its own.

Tip

This will keep in the fridge for 4–5 days, or in the freezer for up to a month.

Tuna sweet potatoes

BEST FOR: A cosy, healthy dinner. To make a veggie version, replace the tuna with an ABC salad – raw grated apple, beetroot and carrot.

SERVES: 2

2 sweet potatoes

160g (6oz) can tuna, drained

1 spring onion, finely chopped

½ red chilli, finely chopped

a handful of cherry tomatoes, halved

a drizzle of olive oil

150g (5oz) cheese of your choice (i.e. goat's cheese, feta, Cheddar)

sea salt and freshly ground black pepper, to taste

Preheat the oven to 180°C/350°F/gas mark 4. Wash and prick the potatoes all over, then place in the oven for 45 minutes or until they're soft inside.

In a bowl, mix the tuna with the spring onion and chilli.

Place the cherry tomatoes on a baking tray, drizzle with a little oil and sprinkle with a pinch of salt and black pepper. Roast for 5-10 minutes until they soften (but don't blacken), then stir into the tuna mixture.

Split open the cooked sweet potatoes and top with the tuna mixture. Sprinkle with the cheese and serve immediately.

My everyday salad dressing

BEST FOR: All your favourite salads. I love to make a batch of this super-simple dressing and keep it in the fridge (it stores for at least a week). It'll need a shake just before you use it.

MAKES: About 180ml

60ml (4 tablespoons) apple cider vinegar

120ml (½ cup) cold-pressed olive oil

1 teaspoon maple syrup or clear honey

1 teaspoon wholegrain mustard

2 garlic cloves, finely chopped

sea salt and freshly ground black pepper, to taste

Place all the ingredients in a jar, screw the lid on and shake to mix together thoroughly.

Store in the fridge until needed.

Sunflower seed and veggie burgers

BEST FOR: These burgers are super versatile and you can really have fun with mixing and matching your vegetables and beans or grains and seasonings as you really can't go wrong, whatever you put in them. Experiment with these three things (any grain or bean, a mix of vegetables, seasoning of your choice) to find your perfect combination.

SERVES: 4–6

140g (1 cup) sunflower seeds
1 teaspoon coconut oil
1 onion, diced
2 garlic cloves, finely chopped
2.5cm (1 in) piece of ginger, grated
1 sweet potato, peeled and diced
1 carrot, peeled and diced
1 stick of celery, diced
½ teaspoon ground turmeric
½ teaspoon ground cumin
½ teaspoon dried coriander
160g (1 cup) cooked rice or quinoa
juice of 1 lemon
salad leaves, to serve

Preheat the oven to 180°C/350°F/gas mark 4.

Place the sunflower seeds in a food processor and blitz until finely chopped.

In a large, heavy-based saucepan, heat the oil and sauté the onion, garlic and ginger until softened but not browned. Add the sweet potato, carrot and celery and stir together with the turmeric, cumin and coriander. Add a splash of water and gently heat for 3–4 minutes until soft but not brown.

Add the rice or quinoa to the pan along with the lemon juice and stir to coat.

Transfer the mixture to the food processor and blend really well with the sunflower seeds.

Using your hands, form the mixture into 4–6 patties, and fry in a little coconut oil in a pan for about 3–4 minutes on each side until golden brown. Serve with a big fresh salad.

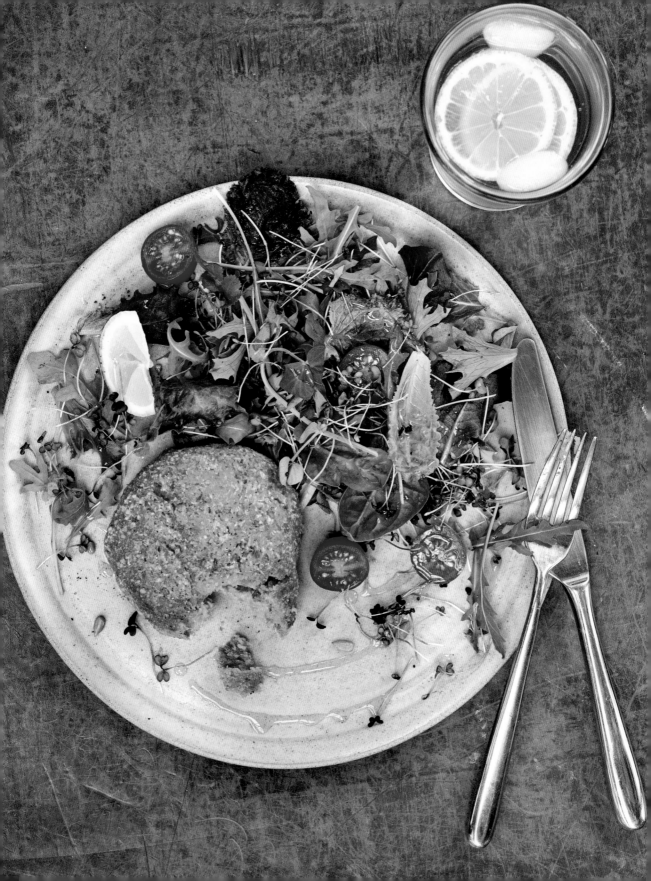

My favourite drinks

PEPPERMINT TEA: This is great for improving your digestion. I'll often make this for myself with either teabags or fresh mint and either boiling hot or cold water.

CUCUMBER AND MINT-INFUSED WATER: If you find water boring, throw in a couple of slices of cucumber and some torn mint leaves. The cucumber tastes deliciously refreshing and also removes harmful toxins from your body.

MORNING SMOOTHIE: 1 scoop of protein powder, ½ banana, a little bit of ice, ¼ avocado, a cup of non-dairy milk, 1 tablespoon of cacao powder and 1 teaspoon of maca powder. Blitz in a blender until smooth. Like it less thick? Add more liquid.

Tip

If my bananas begin to go brown, I peel them, put them in the freezer and use them for my smoothies.

Almond energy balls

BEST FOR: Quick on the go snacks or an afternoon protein pick-me-up.
MAKES: About 10

70g (½ cup) blanched almonds or Brazil nuts

2 tablespoons coconut oil

2 tablespoons maple syrup

2 tablespoons cacao powder

4 tablespoons almond butter

200g (1½ cups) dried apricots, chopped

40g (½ cup) desiccated coconut

Place the nuts in a food processor and roughly chop.

Place all the remaining ingredients, except the coconut, in a large bowl. Add the nuts and mix together thoroughly. Place this mixture in the fridge to firm up for 15 minutes.

Using clean hands, roll the mixture into about 10 small balls, then roll each ball in the coconut to coat.

Store in the fridge until ready to eat. They will keep for 5 days.

Tip

I like to keep my energy balls in the freezer as they last longer and I'm not tempted to pop one in my mouth every time I open the fridge door!

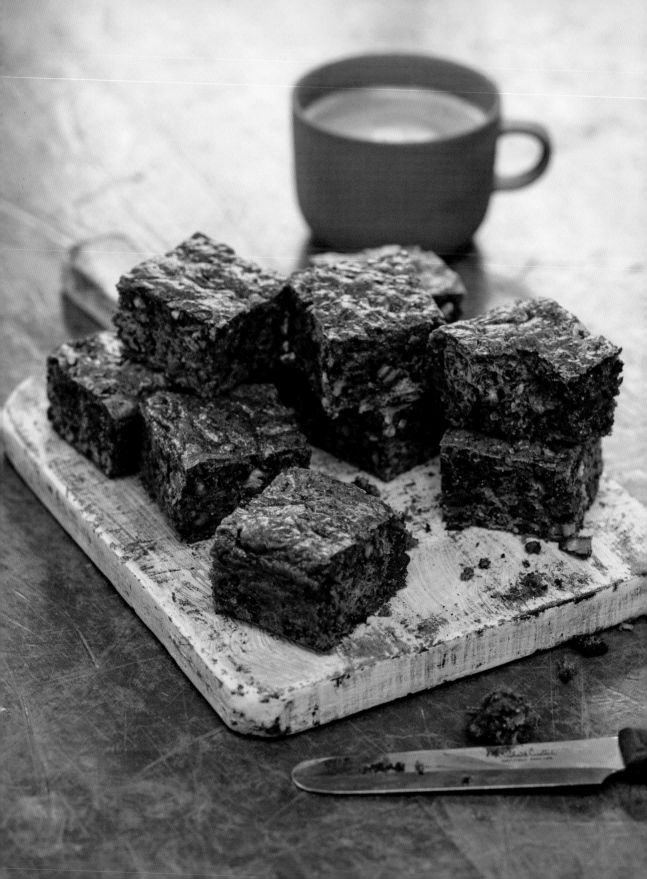

No fuss chocolate brownies

BEST FOR: A simple sweet treat, perfect for afternoon tea.

MAKES: 16

coconut oil, for greasing

1 large courgette, grated

225g (1 cup) almond butter

1 egg, beaten

½ teaspoon vanilla extract

50g (½ cup) pecans, finely chopped

4 tablespoons maple syrup

1 teaspoon ground cinnamon

1 teaspoon bicarbonate of soda

100g (¾ cup) 85- or 90-per cent cocoa dark chocolate, roughly chopped

Preheat the oven to 180°C/350°F/gas mark 4. Grease a 20cm (8 in) square baking tin with a little coconut oil.

In a large bowl, mix together all the remaining ingredients, then pour into the prepared tin and bake for 35 minutes until lightly crusted on top.

Leave to cool, then turn out of the tin and cut into 16 brownie-sized squares.

Tip

I'm a chocoholic and find it hard to go a day without at least a couple of squares of dark chocolate, but I always pick one that's 90% cocoa. As the chocolate taste is very rich and intense, I find that you only need a small amount, plus the dark chocolate contains less sugar than many of the milkier ones. I always advise clients to start increasing the percentage of their chocolate because good nutrition isn't about going without your favourite treats, but rather about moderation and picking the best quality.

Coconut crumble

BEST FOR: When only something sweet will do, this is guaranteed to hit the spot. You can have this crumble hot or cold, for pudding or for breakfast. Also, because fruit is naturally sweet and easily digested it provides a quick blast of energy.

SERVES: 2

350g (12 oz) mixed fruit (my favourites are pears, apples and blackberries)

½ teaspoon ground cinnamon

2 tablespoons flaked almonds, toasted, for sprinkling

2 tablespoons coconut flakes, toasted, for sprinkling

Wash and chop the fruit into chunks (although if using berries, keep them whole). Discard any stones, pips or stems, but leave the peel on for extra nutrients.

Place the fruit in a large saucepan and add roughly 2 tablespoons of water (this prevents the fruit from burning). Cover the pan and gently simmer the fruit over a medium heat until the fruit has softened and broken down, around 3–5 minutes, stirring occasionally.

Once the fruit has softened, remove the lid and stir in the cinnamon.

Divide the fruit between bowls and sprinkle with sliced almonds and coconut flakes. Serve with coconut yogurt or Greek yogurt.

Tip

This is also a great option for breakfast, so if you have any leftovers enjoy them in the morning!

Apple cake

BEST FOR: Sharing with friends or taking on a hike for a picnic.
SERVES: 12

3 eating apples,
cored and diced

250g (2½ cups) ground almonds

2 teaspoons ground cinnamon

½ teaspoon baking powder

3 eggs

a large handful blackberries, plus
extra to serve

a handful of flaked almonds
(optional)

coconut yogurt, to serve (optional)

Preheat the oven to 180°C/350°F/gas mark 4. Line a 20 x 30cm (8 x 10in) tin with baking parchment.

In a large bowl, stir the apples, almonds, cinnamon and baking powder together until all the apples are coated in the mixture.

Beat the eggs and blackberries together in a separate bowl, then slowly add to the apple mixture.

Pour the cake mixture into the prepared tin and sprinkle with flaked almonds, if liked. Bake for 45 minutes, or until firm but still springy to the touch.

Leave to cool, then turn out and cut into slices. Serve with a handful of fresh berries or a dollop of coconut yogurt, if liked.

WORKOUT SUMMARIES

These at-a glance summaries list all the exercises that make up each workout, including reps and timings. When you're more familiar with the movements, it's a quick and easy way to remember the order.

WARMING UP (pages 22–28)
6 minute warm up

Walking Lunges – 60 seconds
Inch Worm – 60 seconds
Downward Dog Heel Paddle – 60 seconds
Catcher Squat to Stand – 60 seconds
Plank to Lunge Rotation – 60 seconds
Low Side-to-Side Lunge – 60 seconds

POSTURE WARM UP (pages 29–35)
5 minute warm up

Shoulder Mobilisation – 10 reps
Cat and Cow – 10 reps
Thoracic Rotation – 5 reps each side
Thread the Needle – 5 reps each side
Wide Squat Twist – 10 reps
Wall Angels – 10 reps

COOLING DOWN (pages 40–45)
6 minute cool down

Standing Shoulder Stretch – 30 second hold
Tricep Stretch With Lean – 30 second hold each side
Lying Hamstring Stretch – 30 second hold each side
Lying Spinal Twist – 30 second hold each side

Pigeon Pose – 30 second hold each side
World's Greatest Stretch – 10 reps each side, hold for 2 seconds each time

----

GET LIVELY IN THE LIVING ROOM (pages 50–55)
Three rounds | 4 minutes per round

No-Rope Skipping – 30 seconds
Sofa Squat with a Loop Band – 10 reps
Sofa Lunge (Right) – 10 reps
Sofa Lunge (Left) – 10 reps
Sofa Reach – 10 reps
Sofa Squat Thrust – 20 reps
Sofa Glute Bridge – 10 reps
Repeat from top.

QUICK KITCHEN WORKOUT (pages 56–61)
Three rounds | 5 minutes per round

Bird-dog – 30 seconds each side
Hip-Hinge With Tea Towel Reach – 30 seconds
Overhead Wide Squat With Side Bends – 30 seconds
Bent Over Row With Tea Towel – 30 seconds
Back Extension With Reach – 30 seconds
Dead Bug – 30 seconds
Repeat from top.

FULL BODY BLAST (pages 66–71)

Three rounds | 6 minutes per round

Reverse Lunge with Knee Drive (left) – 30 seconds

Reverse Lunge with Knee Drive (right) – 30 seconds

Rest 15 seconds

Burpee to Squat – 30 seconds

Rest 15 seconds

Side Lunge Knee Raise (left) – 30 seconds

Side Lunge Knee Raise (right) – 30 seconds

Rest 15 seconds

Plank Toe Taps to Mountain Climber – 30 seconds

Rest 15 seconds

Narrow Squat Wide Squat Lunge Jump Switch – 30 seconds

Rest 15 seconds

Single Leg Balance (left) – 30 seconds

Single Leg Balance (right) – 30 seconds

Repeat from top.

BODY BENCH WORKOUT (pages 72–77)

Three rounds | 4 minutes per round

If you're a beginner or you're short of time, do 3 rounds. If you're an intermediate, or have more time to spare try 4, and if you're advanced and feeling fit, go for 5 rounds.

Bench Squat Jumps – 10 reps

Bench Dips – 10 reps

Bench Mountain Climbers – 10 reps each side

Bench Step-Ups – 10 reps each side

Slow Seated Abs – 10 reps

Bench Press-Ups – 10 reps

Repeat from top.

KILLER KETTLEBELL WORKOUT
(pages 84–89)

Three rounds | 8–10 minutes per round

Ideally, don't rest until the end but, if you need to, take a little rest between each one. If you have more time or want a challenge, repeat 4 or 5 times.

Goblet Squat Press – 10 reps

Kettlebell Swing – 15 reps

Single Leg Deadlift – 10 reps

Lunge and Rotate – 10 reps each side

One Arm Row – 10 reps each side

One Arm Floor Press – 10 reps each side

Rest for 1 minute and drink some water. Repeat from top.

DUMBBELL DYNAMO (pages 90–95)

Three rounds | 6 minutes per round

Ideally, don't rest until the end but, if you need to, take a little rest between each one. If you have more time or want a challenge, repeat 4 or 5 times.

Front Squat – 10 reps

Renegade Row – 10 reps each side

Burpee Squat to Shoulder Press – 10 reps

Bent Over Row to Deadlift – 10 reps

Overhead Pull to Sit Up – 10 reps

Fly With Tabletop Abs – 10 reps

Rest for 1 minute and drink some water. Repeat from top.

STRENGTHEN & LENGTHEN
(pages 100–105)
Two rounds | 6–8 minutes per round

Bear Squat – 5 reps
Yoga Squat – 10 reps
Balance to Warrior Three – 10 reps
each side
Three-Legged Dog to Tiger Curl – 5 reps
each side
Reverse Tabletop – 5 reps, hold for three
breaths each time
Kneeling Side Plank Leg Lift – 10 reps
each side
Repeat from the top.

INNER CORE FOCUS (106–111)
Two rounds | 6–8 minutes per round

Single Leg Bridge – 10 reps each side
Double Leg Stretch – 10 reps
Plank Rotation – 5 reps each side
Donkey Kick (10 reps each side)
Seated Triceps Dips – 10 reps
Bicycles – 10 reps
Repeat from the top.

SUNSHINE WORKOUT (pages 116–123)
Two rounds | 8–10 minutes per round
*If you want more of a challenge, miss out the
rests.*

Skip – 30 seconds
Rest 15 seconds
Sundial Lunge (left) – 30 seconds
Sundial Lunge (right) – 30 seconds
Skip – 30 seconds
Rest 15 seconds
Crab toe touch – 30 seconds
Skip – 30 seconds
Rest 15 seconds
Prone swimming 30 seconds
Skip – 30 seconds
Rest 15 seconds
Plank push ups 30 seconds
Skip – 30 seconds
Rest 15 seconds
Tummy tightener 30 seconds
Repeat from top.

KICK IT WORKOUT (124–129)
Two rounds | 5 minutes per round

Shadow Boxing 30 seconds
Squat to Sidekick (left) – 30 seconds
Squat to Sidekick (right) – 30 seconds
Plank Punch 30 seconds
Back Lunge to Front Kick (left) – 30 seconds
Back Lunge to Front Kick (right) – 30 seconds
Side Sweeps 30 seconds
Slow Roundhouse Kick (left) – 30 seconds
Slow Roundhouse Kick (right) – 30 seconds
Repeat from top.

WORKOUT PLANS

As nice as it is to exercise for pleasure rather than putting pressure on yourself to do it, it's always a good idea to plan so that you have a rough idea of how your week's workouts will pan out. Of course, things can change, but if you have a rough plan in place, you're more likely to fit in your exercise.

TIPS FOR PLANNING YOUR WORKOUTS

- **Take the time to plan properly.** Sit down with your diary once a week and spend 10 minutes working out where you can slot in your workouts. By doing this, you'll make your workouts a priority.
- **Be realistic.** If you plan out way more exercise than you have the time or energy for, you'll end up frustrated and disheartened. It's better to fit in three actual workouts a week than five imaginary ones.
- **Give yourself adequate rest.** If you overdo it, you risk injury – or simply getting tired out. Rest is as important as working out, so remember to give yourself a rest day when you need it.
- **Variety is key.** Don't do exactly the same workout, day in, day out. Chances are you'll quickly grow bored of it and won't feel motivated. Keeping it varied will also keep challenging your body.
- **Learn what you love.** As you try out different kinds of exercise, you'll discover which ones work best for you. Make sure this is reflected in your workout plan.
- **Stay positive.** Congratulate yourself for what you have achieved rather than berating yourself for the targets you might miss.

On the next pages, I've included a couple of sample week-long workout plans to get you started. Everyone's different, so these might not work for you, but they're a starting point.

A normal working week

This plan's focus is motivation and variety. It's tailored around a Monday–Friday, 9–5 working week and includes something different each day so that your workout is something to look forward to rather than a chore.

A super busy week

This is for those weeks where we feel like we have no time to spare, whether we're drowning in deadlines at work or juggling childcare or study. Exercise is often one of the first things to fall by the wayside, but try to make it a priority – even a few minutes will make a huge difference. Think about your time drains (page 12) and drop some of them in favour of a 20-minute workout.

Because most of these workouts aren't really intensive, a rest day isn't strictly needed, but I've factored one in to give you a bit of leeway. Save time and stay motivated by getting overnight oats ready the night before and laying out your gym kit so it's the first thing you see when you wake up.

A normal working week

MONDAY

GYM – DUMBBELL WORKOUT

Beat the Monday blues! Exercise is a mood booster and this will get you set up for a week full of energy and enthusiasm. You can either get up earlier and hit the gym first thing, or swing by after work – whatever fits in best with your schedule.

Warm up (pages 22–38)
Dumbbell Dynamo (pages 90–95)
Cool down (pages 40–45)

TUESDAY

RUN

Whether it's a run, a jog or even a brisk walk, do whatever you can manage. I love to run outside, but you can go for a treadmill if you prefer. Prep a great playlist and really go for it.

Ease into it for the first 5 minutes – this will act as your warm up.
Run/jog for 30 minutes – slow to a walk when you need to
Cool down (pages 40–45)

WEDNESDAY

TRY SOMETHING NEW

Get out of your comfort zone and try a new class. Sometimes this can be intimidating, so take measures to make sure you don't back out – sign up in advance or go with a friend. Make sure you choose something that fits in with your regular schedule so that if you enjoy it, you can go each week. .

THURSDAY

TAKE IT OUTSIDE – BENCH WORKOUT

Get outside into the fresh air. New surroundings, clean air and the endorphin hit of a workout will leave you feeling excellent.

Warm up (pages 22–38)
Body Bench workout (pages 72–77)
Cool down (pages 40–45)

FRIDAY

REST DAY

Just because it's a rest day, doesn't mean you can't be active. Take the stairs, get off the bus a stop early and walk, stand up and pace whenever you're on the phone. Just move more and sit less – that's non-exercise activity thermogenesis, or NEAT.

SATURDAY

GYM – KETTLEBELL WORKOUT

This is a strength building workout that will leave you feeling motivated and powerful. If you don't have/want a gym membership, you can buy a kettlebell or dumbbells and do this at home. However, I do recommend you give the gym a try – it's a great atmosphere.

Warm up (pages 22–38)
Kettlebell Killer Workout (pages 84–89)
Cool down (pages 40–45)

SUNDAY

WALK

If you prefer, you can go for another run today, but Sunday is the perfect day to take a walk with family and friends.

If you like, you can incorporate some stretches from the cool down (pages 40–45).

A super busy week

MONDAY

AT HOME – SOFA WORKOUT

Set your alarm 25 minutes earlier than normal and start your day with this living room workout. You can complete it while the kids are having breakfast or while you're catching up on the morning news.

Warm up (pages 22–38)
Get Lively in the Living Room (pages 50–55 – only two rounds)
Cool down (pages 40–45 – pick two stretches)

TUESDAY

TAKE THE STAIRS

Today, commit to making the most of your NEAT. Stay away from lifts and escalators! Take the stairs, walk to work if you can (or get off the bus a stop early if you can't) and make sure you're moving around whenever you're on the phone. I'm not counting this as a rest day because I really want you to focus on moving as much as possible.

WEDNESDAY

STUDIO – YOGA WORKOUT

You can complete this one at home, so you don't have to lose any time travelling to the gym or studio. Again, set your alarm a little earlier than usual. Or, if you're not a morning person, do this in the early evening – it makes a great full stop at the end of a working day before you wind down for the night.

Strengthen & Lengthen (pages 100–105 – two rounds – no need to warm up or cool down)

THURSDAY

HOLIDAY – SUNSHINE WORKOUT

OK, you might need a holiday, but in the middle of a busy week this is the closest you're getting! It's quick and fun and will help to lift your mood.

Warm up (pages 22–38)
Sunshine workout (pages 116–123 – just one round)
Cool down (pages 40–45 – pick two stretches)

FRIDAY

REST DAY

Again, remember your NEAT – keep moving even if you don't have any workouts scheduled in. And if you're spending a long week glued to your desk, remember to do some posture stretches (pages 36–39) to avoid feeling cramped and uncomfortable.

SATURDAY

TAKE IT OUTSIDE – BODY BLAST

If you've had a long, busy week, you really need to get out and loosen up. Hopefully you can find time today to complete a full workout – it'll leave you feeling re-energised and positive. If you don't have time for all three rounds, just do two.

Warm up (pages 22–38)
Full body blast (pages 66–71)

SUNDAY

STUDIO – PILATES

Again, you can do this one at home. There's no warm up or cool down needed. Just fit it in wherever you can – a calming and reflective way to end the week.

Inner Core Focus (pages 106–111)

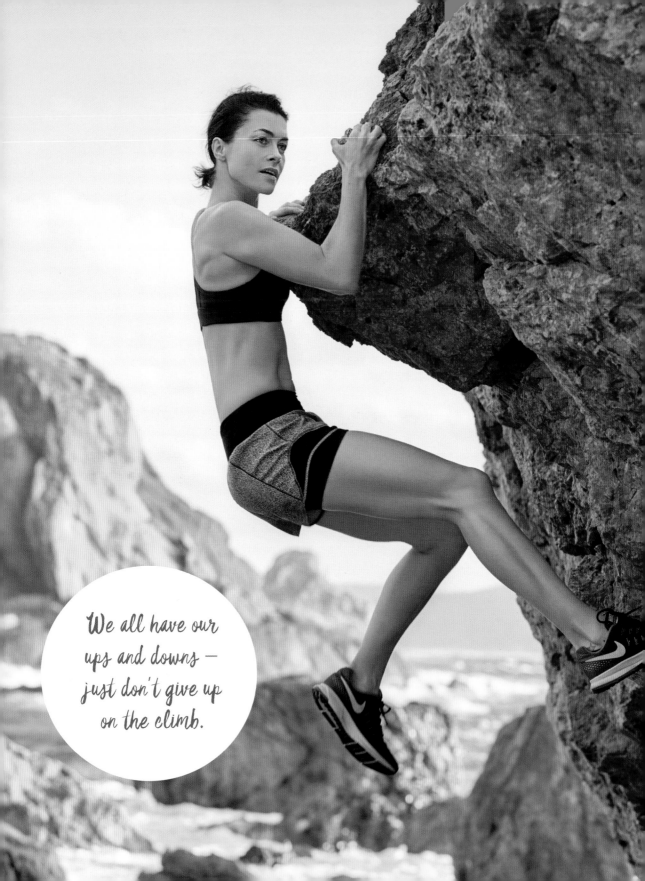

We all have our ups and downs — just don't give up on the climb.

INDEX

ACKNOWLEDGEMENTS

I couldn't have made this book without the support and help of an awesome team behind the scenes. Thank you for all your hard work Chloe Beeney, Patrizia Lio, Tania Gomes, Maria Lally, Mikael Kenta, Kyle Cathie, Vicki Murrell, Victoria Scales, Sarah Kyle and Julia Azzarello.

A special thanks to Tara O'Sullivan, the best editor anyone could hope for, and Sebastian Roos for your exquisite photography.

A huge thanks to all my clients past and present. I am inspired daily by your energy and commitment, each day I work with you all makes my heart smile. Thank you to my clients who contributed their stories and quotes to the book: Amie, Annelies, Claire, Kate, Sienna, Silvia.

And of course, my wonderful family. I love you all so much.

An Hachette UK Company
www.hachette.co.uk

First published in Great Britain in 2018
by Kyle Books, an imprint of Kyle Cathie Ltd
Carmelite House, 50 Victoria Embankment
London EC4Y 0DZ
www.kylebooks.co.uk

10 9 8 7 6 5 4 3 2

ISBN 978 0 85783 446 1

Text © 2018 Holly Davidson
Design © 2018 Kyle Books
Photographs © 2018 Sebastian Roos

Distributed in the US by Hachette Book Group, 1290 Avenue of the Americas, 4th and 5th Floors, New York, NY 10104

Distributed in Canada by Canadian Manda Group, 664 Annette St., Toronto, Ontario, Canada M6S 2C8

Holly Davidson is hereby identified as the author of this work in accordance with Section 77 of the Copyright, Designs and Patents Act 1988.

Project Editor: Tara O'Sullivan
Copy Editor: Vicki Murrell
Editorial Assistant: Sarah Kyle
Designer: Tania Gomes
Photographer: Sebastian Roos
Stylist: Chloe Beeney
Production: Lisa Pinnell

A Cataloguing in Publication record for this title is available from the British Library.

Printed and bound in China

outfits and suppliers

The author and the publishers would like to thank the following brands, who generously provided clothing and equipment for the photo shoots for this book.
Adidas (www.adidas.co.uk)
GapFit (www.gap.co.uk)
Lululemon (www.lululemon.co.uk)
Nike (www.nike.com)
Sweaty Betty (www.sweatybetty.com)
Varley (www.varley.com)
Zatki Active (www.zatkiactive.com)

Cover, page 2, pages 116-123 sports bra and leggings by Varley | Page 6 top by GapFit, shorts by Zatki Active | Pages 8, 21, 35 trousers by Sweaty Betty, top by Lululemon | Pages 11, 62, 80, 83, 124-129, 174 – Hotty Hot Short Naked by Lululemon and sports bra by GapFit | Pages 16 and 66–71 – leggings by Ivy Park, sports bra by GapFit | Pages 22-28 and 84–89 – top by Adidas, Wunder Under High Rise Tights by Lululemon | Pages 29-34 – leggings by Adidas, top by Lululemon | Pages 36-39 – leggings and sports bra by Zatki Active, top by GapFit | Pages 40-45 – trousers by Sweaty Betty, sports bra by Varley | Page 46 – trousers by Sweaty Betty, top by GapFit | Pages 50–55 – leggings and top by Zatki Active | Pages 56–61 – Leggings by GapFit, top by Zatki Active | Page 64 - shorts, top, hat by GapFit | Page 65 – leggings and neck warmer by Zatki Active, gilet and hat by Nike | Pages 72-77 – trousers by Sweaty Betty, sports bra by GapFit | Pages 90–95 – top and leggings by Sweaty Betty | Pages 96, 100–105 – leggings and top by Zatki Active | Page 79, 112, 115, 130 – black and white shorts, black top by GapFit | Pages 99, 106–111 – leggings and top by Ivy Park | Page 135 – Jumper by Gap | All shoes by Nike